OPTIC NERVE

Edited by **Felicia M. Ferreri**

Optic Nerve
http://dx.doi.org/10.5772/intechopen.72958
Edited by Felicia M. Ferreri

Contributors

José M. Ramírez, Ana I. Ramírez, Juan J Salazar, Rosa De Hoz, Elena Salobrar-Garcia, José A Fernández-Albarral, Inés López-Cuenca, Pilar Rojas, Alberto Triviño, Blanca Rojas, Daniah Alshowaeir, Tariq Al-Zahem, Hind Alkatan, Bilyana Mihaylova, Galina Dimitrova, Lawan Abdu, Marija Radenkovic, Andi Arus Victor, Felicia M. Ferreri

First published in London, United Kingdom, 2019 by IntechOpen
IntechOpen is the global imprint of INTECHOPEN LIMITED, registered in England and Wales, registration number: 11086078, The Shard, 25th floor, 32 London Bridge Street
London, SE19SG – United Kingdom
Printed in Croatia

British Library Cataloguing-in-Publication Data
A catalogue record for this book is available from the British Library

Additional hard copies can be obtained from orders@intechopen.com

Optic Nerve, Edited by Felicia M. Ferreri
p. cm.
Print ISBN 978-1-78984-966-0
Online ISBN 978-1-78984-967-7

For EU product safety concerns:
IN TECH d.o.o., Prolaz Marije Krucifikse Kozulić 3, 51000 Rijeka, Croatia,
info@intechopen.com or visit our website at intechopen.com.

Meet the editor

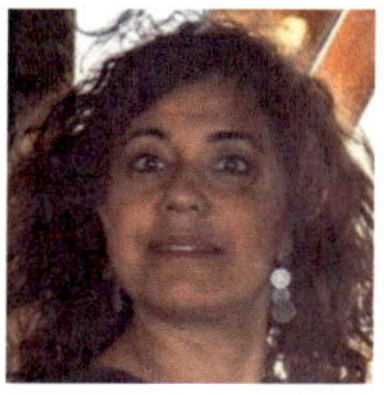

Felicia M. Ferreri graduated summa cum laude from the University of Messina, Italy, in 1998 and completed her ophthalmology residency at the Policlinico Universitario, Messina, in 2002. She was interned at San Raffaele Hospital in Milan (corneal section) and at the Hospital Careggi in Florence (pediatric ophthalmology diseases). She spent research periods in Seville (Virginio del Rocio Hospital), Madrid (San Carlos Hospital), Manchester (Bolton Hospital), and Rio de Janiero (Universidade Fluminense).

She has served as coinvestigator for many national and international clinical trials. Since 2002, she has been an assistant professor in ophthalmology at the University of Messina. Her research interests are in the areas of glaucoma, neuro-ophthalmology, pediatric ophthalmology, and cataract. She has authored more than 50 scientific papers.

Contents

Preface IX

Section 1 **Anatomy of the Optic Nerve and Anomalies in its Development 1**

Chapter 1 **Introductory Chapter: The Dysthyroid Optic Neuropathy 3**
Felicia M. Ferreri and Giuseppina Ferreri

Chapter 2 **Anatomy of the Human Optic Nerve: Structure and Function 11**
Juan J. Salazar, Ana I. Ramírez, Rosa De Hoz, Elena Salobrar-Garcia, Pilar Rojas, José A. Fernández-Albarral, Inés López-Cuenca, Blanca Rojas, Alberto Triviño and José M. Ramírez

Chapter 3 **Optic Nerve: Developmental Anomalies and Common Tumors 57**
Hind Alkatan, Daniah Alshowaeir and Tariq Alzahem

Chapter 4 **Optic Nerve Changes in Diabetic Retinopathy 85**
Andi Arus Victor

Section 2 **Clinical Challenges in Optic Nerve Disorder Management 105**

Chapter 5 **Evaluation of Retinal Nerve Fiber Layer and Inner Macular Layers in Primary Open-Angle Glaucoma with Spectral-Domain Optical Coherence Tomography 107**
Bilyana Mihaylova and Galina Dimitrova

Chapter 6 **Clinical Assessment of Lesions Compressing the Visual Pathway 125**
Lawan Abdu

Chapter 7 **Contribution to the Optic Nerve 139**
Marija Radenković

Preface

The study of the optic nerve, its structure, functioning, and disorders is a key topic for both researchers and clinicians.

Many pathologies in fact can affect the optic nerve: some of them are congenital (think of myelinated nerve fibers, morning glory syndrome, choristoma, and rare anomalies to name a few), while others can be classified as tumors both in primary form (i.e., if neoplasia surrounds the optic nerve sheath) and secondary form (relevant examples are medulloepithelioma, optic nerve meningioma, and others). Optic nerve examination is arguably the most important component of the evaluation of a glaucoma patient. The appearance of the optic nerve is therefore crucial to diagnose glaucoma and detect its progression.

Due to the variety and complexity of disorders affecting the optic nerve, both researchers and physicians need a comprehensive reference that starts from detailing the anatomy of the optic nerve, illustrates how the most modern diagnostic procedures (think of imaging techniques) can be effectively employed for clinical purposes, and, last but not the least, shows how to manage complex clinical cases that may occur in the daily life of an ophthalmologist.

This book aims to elevate itself as an authoritative reference that can help broad and heterogeneous audiences, ranging from resident students to clinicians, neuroscientists, researchers, and, ultimately, surgeons.

The book is divided into two main sections: it starts by reviewing in detail the anatomy of the optic nerve with special emphasis on the optic nerve head and chiasm. Organization of the optic nerve into regions is explored in detail with a thorough discussion of axoplasmic flow, glial barriers, and the lamina cribrosa.

This book then concentrates on embryology, physiology, and pathology of the optic nerve and introduces clinical features and imaging findings that help clinicians in detecting disorders and making a diagnosis.

The book will explore in detail the relationship between neuroendocrine structures and functional/structural modifications occurring in the optic nerve: a first example is drawn by diabetic retinopathy and we will pay a special attention to changes to the optic nerve it generates such as diabetic papillopathy and neovascularization of the optic disc.

We will also discuss diagnostic tests (e.g., optical coherence tomography and visual evoked potential) that allow us to detect structural and functional changes to the optic nerve.

We will finally shift to analysis of optic nerve head drusen, a class of congenital anomalies that may produce a progressive optic neuropathy but are hard to detect and manage even for the more experienced clinicians.

Felicia M. Ferreri
University of Messina
Messina, Italy

Section 1

Anatomy of the Optic Nerve and Anomalies in its Development

Chapter 1

Introductory Chapter: The Dysthyroid Optic Neuropathy

Felicia M. Ferreri and Giuseppina Ferreri

Additional information is available at the end of the chapter

http://dx.doi.org/10.5772/intechopen.82491

1. Introduction

Graves' orbitopathy—often known as Basedowian ophthalmopathy—is an autoimmune disorder that occurs in 5% of patients affected by the thyroid disease [1].

Graves' orbitopathy (GO) mainly affects retrobulbar soft tissue [2] and it is the extra thyroidal manifestation of Graves' disease and the most common cause of exophthalmos. The GO can have a major impact on the patient life, from both functional and aesthetic point of view; to some extent, it can be considered as an event deeply affecting the quality of life of the patients. The most serious consequence of GO is perhaps the *dysthyroid optic neuropathy (DON)*, which is due to compression caused by the swelling of extraocular muscles and orbital fat [3].

Many studies in the latest two centuries concentrated on GO and its treatments [4]. Ocular changes associated with thyroid disease, in fact, have been described by Graves in 1835 and by Von Basedow in 1840, but they are likely to be observed and studied by Parry in 1786, who published posthumously a paper on GO in 1825.

Despite ongoing advances in basic science and clinical research, the pathogenesis of GO is still unclear and highly effective therapeutic strategies remain elusive. The diagnosis of GO is mainly based on laboratory tests devoted to investigate thyroid dysfunction and/or autoimmunity. Recently, however, imaging approaches (among which we cite computed tomography, magnetic resonance imaging, ultrasound, and colour Doppler imaging) are increasingly adopted both in the diagnosis stage and in the follow-up, after proper clinical or surgical treatments have been applied [5, 6]. Imaging techniques, in particular, are relevant to spot morphological abnormalities affecting the orbital structures as well as to classify early stages of the diseases. In addition, imaging techniques are useful to identify those patients who are likely to get affected from DON in advance; such knowledge is crucial for an early treatment, and on the long run, it is effective in avoiding visual loss.

This chapter mainly focuses on DON, and it aims at illustrating the most recent advances in its diagnosis and treatment. The chapter is structured as follows: we introduce the Graves' orbitopathy, and then, we detail the main features of DON as well as the diagnostic procedures usually followed in clinical practice.

2. The Graves' orbitopathy

Graves' orbitopathy (GO) is the most common extra-thyroidal manifestation of Graves' disease (GD). It roughly occurs in 25–50% of patients who are affected from the GD [4].

GO may occur during or after the onset of hyperthyroidism and less frequently in euthyroid or hypothyroid patients [4].

Some studies highlighted a strong association between immunogenic hyperthyroidism and orbitopathy, which forces us to conjecture that the antigen responsible for these diverse conditions may be shared by the thyroid gland and orbital tissues [7].

GO displays an *active phase* (also called *inflammatory stage*) and an *inactive phase* (also called *fibrotic stage*). In the active phase, we notice, on one hand, an expansion of tissue, which is generally due to inflammation, the accumulation of glycosaminoglycans and an increased fat content; such an expansion is balanced by the space constraint imposed by the bony orbit. The signs and symptoms of the GO during the active stage include lid retraction, proptosis, conjunctival injection, chemosis, diplopia, corneal ulceration, and rarely, disthiroid optic neuropathy (DON), which will be later described.

The active stage length generally varies from 18 to 24 months; such a stage is then followed by an inactive stage, which is mainly characterised by clinical signs such as lid retraction, proptosis, and restrictive strabismus.

The management of patients with GO is challenging, and in the absence of objective evidence of thyroid dysfunction, GO is hard to diagnose [8].

The main clinical features to diagnose GO are discussed in Bartley and Gorman [9]: an effective indicator of GO is when eyelid retraction occurs in association with thyroid dysfunction or abnormal regulation, exophthalmos, optic nerve dysfunction, DON, or extraocular muscle involvement. If eyelid retraction is absent, further laboratory tests are needed.

More recently, magnetic resonance imaging (MRI) has been employed to distinguish the acute inflammatory active disease from fibrotic stage disease [10]. MRI is a mandatory choice in the management of doubtful cases (e.g., asymmetrical orbital involvement), and it is required to exclude any other orbital pathology.

Several classification systems are today available to assess the clinical manifestations of GO. The first one is due to Werner [11], who introduced the so-called NO SPECS classification;

this is an acronym which stands for *No physical signs or symptoms, Only signs, Soft tissue involvement, Proptosis, Extraocular muscle signs, Corneal involvement, and Sight loss.*

NO SPECS classification was subsequently updated, and it is now largely adopted in clinical practice, along with its variants [12]. The modified version of NOSPECS is reported in **Table 1**.

Class	Grade	Suggestion for grading
O		No physical signs or symptoms
I		Only signs
II		Soft tissue involvement
	0	Absent
	a	Minimal
	b	Moderate
	c	Marked
III		Proptosis (3 mm or more of normal upper limits with or without symptoms)
	0	Absent
	a	3 or 4 mm over upper normal
	b	5 to 7 mm increase
	c	8 mm increase
IV		Extraocular muscle involvement (usually with diplopia)
	a	Absent
	b	Limitation of motion at extremes of gaze
	c	Evident restriction of motion
	d	Fixation of a globe or globes
V		Corneal involvement (primarily due to lagophthalmos)
	0	Absent
	a	Stippling of cornea
	b	Ulceration
	c	Clouding, necrosis and perforation
VI		Sight Loss (due to optic nerve involvement)
	0	Absent
	a	Disc pallor or choking, or visual field defect, vision 20/20 or 20/60
	b	The same but vision 20/70–20/200
	c	Blindness, vision less than 20/200

Table 1. NO SPECS modified classification.

NO SPECS classification is conceived to measure the degree of severity of GO, and therefore, it is not suitable to distinguish the active GO stage from the inactive one. This implies that NO SPECS classification allows for identifying a treatment on the basis of the symptom severity rather than on the actual progression of the disease. To this end, Mourits et al. [13] introduced the *Clinical Activity Score (CAS)*, with the goal of discriminating the active from the inactive stage of the disease. CAS table was subsequently updated [14].

3. The dysthyroid optic neuropathy

Dysthyroid optic neuropathy (DON) is the most feared complication of thyroid eye disease, and it constitutes an important factor of permanent or temporary disability.

Fortunately, DON occurs with a low incidence; in fact, some studies estimate that it affects 4–8% of patients affected by thyroid eye disease [15].

Some researchers propose inflammatory [16, 17] and ischemic models [18] to explain DON; however, the most widely accepted explanation is that DON depends on the mechanical compression of the optic nerve at the orbital apex by the enlarged extraocular muscles [19].

The main features to diagnose disthiroid optic neuropathy (DON) are listed below:

1. Impaired colour vision
2. Optic disc swelling/atrophy
3. Abnormal visual acuity
4. Relative afferent pupillary defect
5. Abnormal VEPs
6. Crowded apex on scanning
7. Abnormal visual fields
8. Atrophy of the optic nerve head
9. Edema

Patients with GO are assumed to be affected by DON if at least one of the aforementioned features is present and no other cause for the defect is observed; unfortunately, visual impairment in GO is sometimes linked with other factors, as observed by Dayan and Dayan [20]. This implies that direct optic nerve function testing in GO patients is the source of misleading results which makes a DON diagnosis hard.

The availability of effective clinical tests is of great relevance in DON management: when diagnosed, DON needs urgent treatment with medical (e.g., high dose intravenous methylprednisolone) or surgical decompression (e.g., bone removal decompression) to avoid permanent or progressive visual loss [16]. Kazim et al. [17] analysed a set of five patients in whom the extraocular muscle enlargement was one of the causes of DON, and they proved that orbital fat decompression was an effective alternative to bony decompression.

Treatments above carry a considerable risk of morbidity, and hence, a correct diagnosis is a key ingredient to ensure that those patients affected by DON are treated promptly, while those unaffected are spared the risks associated with treatment.

The diagnosis of GO and DON is based primarily on clinical signs from laboratory test results which aim at detecting thyroid dysfunction and autoimmunity. The visual field along with optical coherence tomography (OCT) provides rich information about DON and its severity. In **Figure 1**, we report the visual field of an individual with a severe DON complication.

More recently, *imaging studies*, such as computed tomography (CT), magnetic resonance imaging (MRI), ultrasonography (US), and colour Doppler imaging (CDI), can also be extremely important in both the diagnosis and clinical or surgical follow-up [3].

Imaging studies are able to analyse extraocular muscle involvement and may help distinguish the early acute inflammatory stage from the fibrotic and inactive stage of the disease [10]. In case of patients prone to develop DON, the extensive usage of imaging approaches makes a timely diagnosis possible, avoiding permanent visual loss.

Giaconi et al. [5] analysed the utility of CT imaging in identifying patients with DON. They found that patients with Graves' orbitopathy who have severe optic nerve crowding, intracranial fat prolapse and/or muscle index greater than 50% present on orbital CT scans are more likely to have coexisting optic neuropathy.

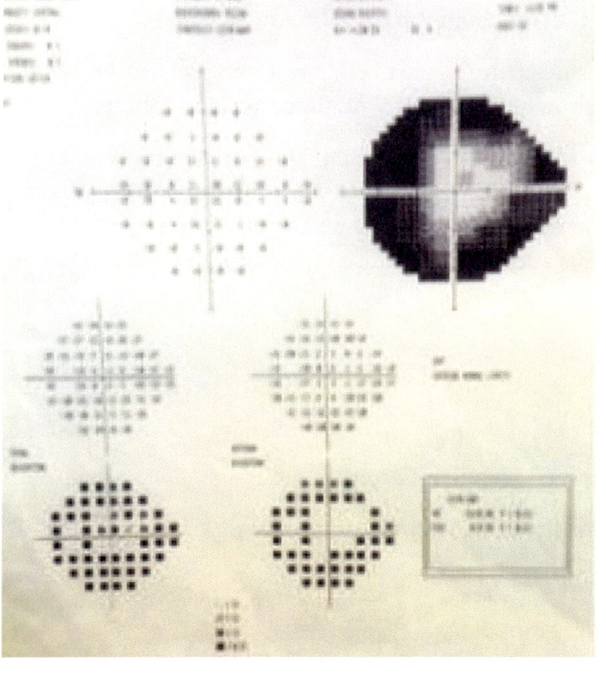

Figure 1. Visual field of a patient with severe DON complication.

An important result to cite is due to Goncalves et al. [3], who targeted at assessing the ability of multi-detector CT to detect DON. The proposed study involved 93 patients who underwent a complete neuro-ophthalmic examination, as well as a CT scan. For each individual, orbital fat and muscle volume were estimated on the basis of their attenuation factors. The authors computed a pair of metrics, namely: *(a) the volumetric crowding index*, defined as the ratio of the soft tissue to the orbital fat volume, and *(b) the volumetric orbital apex crowding index*, which is the ratio of the extraocular muscles to the orbital fat volume. Two groups of orbits (with and without dysthyroid optic neuropathy) were compared.

The main result of such a study was that the orbital volumetric crowding index was the most effective predictor of dysthyroid optic neuropathy in comparison with the previously described computed tomography indexes.

4. Conclusions

This chapter targets at describing the main features of the dysthyroid optic neuropathy (DON), one of the most severe complications of Graves' syndrome.

We first described the clinical signs and test laboratory, which are commonly used to diagnose DON. We also focused on modern imaging techniques such as ultrasonography and magnetic resonance which represent one of the most promising tools that ophthalmologist can use to promptly diagnose DON. There are in fact only few studies on small groups of patients revealing the high potential of imaging techniques and their ability to overcome the common drawbacks that the laboratory test incurs.

We believe that, in the near future, we need to test imaging techniques on large samples to get a more accurate assessment of their potentialities and limitations.

A lot of work is still needed in the field of DON treatments: in fact, only steroid drugs (methylprednisolone) are commonly used, and from a surgical standpoint, the only available therapeutic options are bone and fat compression. A novel and important research avenue is the study of effective surgical procedures which can actually improve the quality of life of patients.

Author details

Felicia M. Ferreri[1]* and Giuseppina Ferreri[2]

*Address all correspondence to: fferreri@unime.it

1 University of Messina, Italy

2 Hospital Sesto S. Giovanni, Italy

References

[1] Sabetti L, Serra MG, Furcese N, Baschieri I, Balestrazzi E. Basedowian ophthalmopathy: Diagnostic criteria and new therapeutical prospectives. In: Ultrasonography in Ophthalmology XV. Springer; 1997. pp. 347-353

[2] Saraci G, Treta A. Ocular changes and approaches of ophthalmopathy in Basedow-Graves-Parry-Flajani disease. Maedica. 2011;**6**(2):146

[3] Gonçalves ACP, Silva LN, Gebrim EMMS, Matayoshi S, Monteiro MLR. Predicting dysthyroid optic neuropathy using computed tomography volumetric analyses of orbital structures. Clinics. 2012;**67**(8):891-896

[4] Bahn RS. Graves' ophthalmopathy. New England Journal of Medicine. 2010;**362**(8):726-738

[5] Giaconi JA, Kazim M, Rho T, Pfaff C. CT scan evidence of dysthyroid optic neuropathy. Ophthalmic Plastic & Reconstructive Surgery. 2002;**18**(3):177-182

[6] Kahaly GJ. Imaging in thyroid-associated orbitopathy. European Journal of endocrinology. 2001;**145**(2):107-118

[7] Heufelder AE. Pathogenesesis of ophthalmopathy in autoimmune thyroid disease. Reviews in Endocrine & Metabolic Disorders. 2000;**1**(1-2):87-95

[8] Feldon S. Graves' ophthalmopathy: Is it really thyroid disease? Archives of Internal Medicine. 1990;**150**(5):948-950

[9] Bartley GB, Gorman CA. Diagnostic criteria for Graves' ophthalmopathy. American Journal of Ophthalmology. 1995;**119**(6):792-795

[10] Kirsch E, von Arx G, Hammer B. Imaging in Graves' orbitopathy. Orbit. 2009;**28**(4):219-225

[11] Werner S. Classification of the eye changes of Graves' disease. American Journal of Ophthalmology. 1969;**68**(4):646-648

[12] Werner S. Modification of the classification of the eye changes of Graves' disease. American Journal of Ophthalmology. 1977;**83**(5):725-727

[13] Mourits MPH, Koornneef L, Wiersinga WM, Prummel MF, Berghout A, Van Der Gaag R. Clinical criteria for the assessment of disease activity in Graves' ophthalmopathy: A novel approach. British Journal of Ophthalmology. 1989;**73**(8):639-644

[14] Mourits MP, Prummel MF, Wiersinga WM, Koornneef L. Clinical activity score as a guide in the management of patients with Graves' ophthalmopathy. Clinical Endocrinology. 1997;**47**(1):9-14

[15] Bartley GB. The epidemiologic characteristics and clinical course of ophthalmopathy associated with autoimmune thyroid disease in Olmsted county, Minnesota. Transactions of the American Ophthalmological Society. 1994;**92**:477

[16] Trobe JD, Glaser JS, Laflamme P. Dysthyroid optic neuropathy: Clinical profile and rationale for management. Archives of Ophthalmology. 1978;**96**(7):1199-1209

[17] Kazim M, Trokel SL, Acaroglu G, Elliott A. Reversal of dysthyroid optic neuropathy following orbital fat decompression. British Journal of Ophthalmology. 2000;**84**(6):600-605

[18] Dosso A, Safran AB, Sunaric G, Burger A. Anterior ischemic optic neuropathy in Graves' disease. Journal of neuro-ophthalmology: The Official Journal of the North American Neuro-Ophthalmology Society. 1994;**14**(3):170-174

[19] Feldon SE, Muramatsu S, Weiner JM. Clinical classification of Graves' ophthalmopathy: Identification of risk factors for optic neuropathy. Archives of Ophthalmology. 1984; **102**(10):1469-1472

[20] Dayan CM, Dayan MR. Dysthyroid optic neuropathy: A clinical diagnosis or a definable entity?; 2007

Chapter 2

Anatomy of the Human Optic Nerve: Structure and Function

Juan J. Salazar, Ana I. Ramírez, Rosa De Hoz,
Elena Salobrar-Garcia, Pilar Rojas,
José A. Fernández-Albarral, Inés López-Cuenca,
Blanca Rojas, Alberto Triviño and José M. Ramírez

Additional information is available at the end of the chapter

http://dx.doi.org/10.5772/intechopen.79827

Abstract

The optic nerve (ON) is constituted by the axons of the retinal ganglion cells (RGCs). These axons are distributed in an organized pattern from the soma of the RGC to the lateral geniculated nucleus (where most of the neurons synapse). The key points of the ON are the optic nerve head and chiasm. This chapter will include a detailed and updated review of the ON different parts: RGC axons, glial cells, connective tissue of the lamina cribrosa and the septum and the blood vessels derivate from the central retina artery and from the ciliary system. There will be an up-to-date description about the superficial nerve fibre layer, including their organization, and about prelaminar, laminar and retrolaminar regions, emphasizing the axoplasmic flow, glial barriers, biomechanics of the lamina cribrosa and the role of the macro- and microglia in their working.

Keywords: optic nerve, lamina cribrosa, prelaminar region, retrolaminar region, vascularization, glioarchitecture, blood barrier

1. Introduction

The retina and the optic nerve constitute the beginning of the visual pathway. The visual pathway is made up, in addition to the retina and optic nerves (ON), of the optic chiasma, optic tracts, lateral geniculate nucleus (LGN), optic radiations and visual cortex. There are other areas of the cortex also associated with vision such as the frontal eye fields [1–4].

1.1. Retina

Apart from the cells of association (the horizontal cells and amacrine cells) and glial cells (the Müller cells, astrocytes and microglia), the retina is composed of three superimposed neurons that establish a connection with each other. The external neuron is the photoreceptor. The second neuron, the bipolar cell, is in the nuclear layer. The third or internal neuron is the ganglion cell (GC) [1]. The cell bodies of most of the GCs are located in the ganglion cell layer (GCL), between the retinal nerve fibre layer (NFL) and the inner plexiform layer [2]. Their axons form the retinal NFL and synapse with neurons in the LGN of the thalamus [1, 2]. There are up to seven layers of GC bodies in the central retina or fovea (60–80 μm thickness) and a few as one cell layer in the peripheral retina (10–20 μm) [2]. There are between 500.000 and 1.2 million GCs per retina [1, 4] and approximately 100 rods and 4–6 cones per GC [2].

The axons form criss-crossed bundles but are separated and ensheathed by glial cells [1, 2]. The bundles leave the eye to form the optic nerve (ON). Upon existing through the lamina cribrosa, the axons become myelinated with oligodendrocytes [1, 2].

The visual field (VF) and the retina have an inverted and reversed relationship. The upper VF falls on the inferior retina (below the fovea), lower VF on the superior retina, nasal VF on the temporal retina and temporal VF on the nasal retina [3].

One of the most commonly used diagnostic tests in ophthalmology is the optic coherence tomography (OCT). This test analyses the ganglion cell complex (GCC) which represents the combination of three layers: the NFL, GCL and inner plexiform layer. These layers contain, respectively, the axons, the cell bodies and the dendrites of the ganglion cells.

1.2. Optic nerve

The ON is formed by the convergence of GC axons at the optic disc or papilla. In the papilla there are no photoreceptors, and it represents the blind spot [1]. Foveal/macular fibres constitute around 90% of all axons leaving the eye and forming the papillomacular bundle [2].

The optic nerve has some characteristics that make it unique. It is the only tract in the central nervous system (CNS) to leave the cranial cavity and the only one that can be visualized clinically. It is subdivided into fascicles by connective tissue and glial septa, and it is surrounded by cerebrospinal fluid [2].

The ON can be divided into four main portions (**Figure 1**):

- Intraocular nerve head (1 mm in length) (**Figures 2** and **3A**)

It extends from the surface of the optic disc to the posterior margins of the sclera. The nerve fibres are not myelinated in this portion. Myelination commences approximately with the termination of the subarachnoid space at the posterior limits of lamina cribrosa [1, 2] (**Figures 3F1** and **F2**).

- Intraorbital (25–30 mm)

http://dx.doi.org/10.5772/intechopen.79827

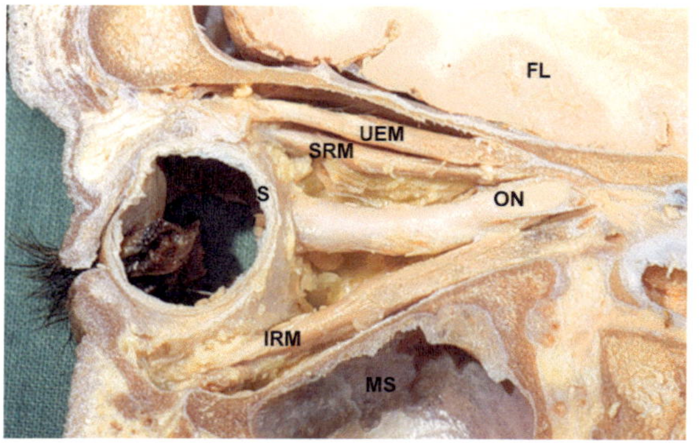

Figure 1. Human optic nerve. Parasagittal cut at the level of the orbit. The intraorbital path of the optic nerve (ON), surrounded by the retrobulbar fat and the extrinsic eye muscles, is observed (FL, frontal lobe; IRM, inferior rectus muscle; MS, maxillary sinus; S, sclera; SRM, superior rectus muscle; UEM, upper eyelid muscle). *Provided by Mérida JR from Desarrollo del nervio Optico in Neuropatias ópticas diagnóstico y tratamiento. Industria Grafica Mae Spain, 2002, p13.*

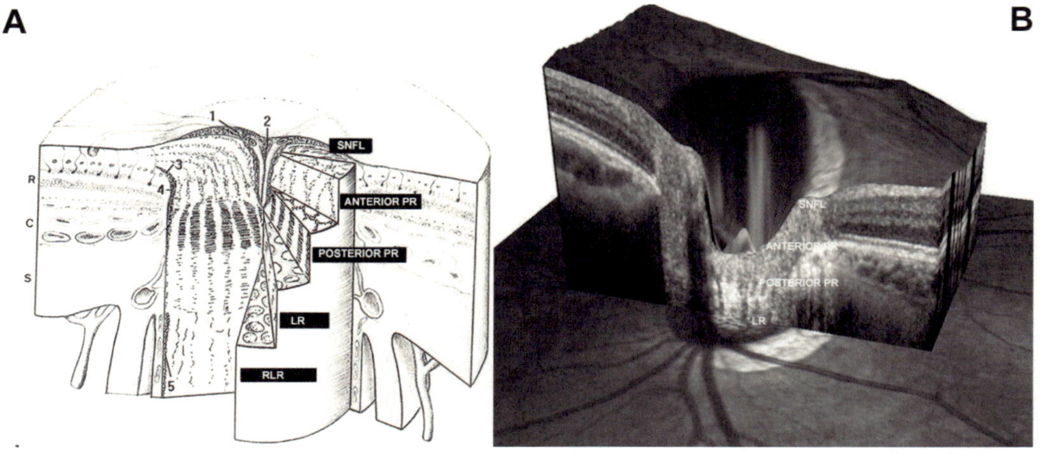

Figure 2. Optic nerve head (ONH). (A) Three-dimensional scheme of the optic nerve head (ONH) regions. (1) Elschnig internal limiting membrane, (2) Kuhnt central meniscus, (3) Kuhnt intermediary tissue, (4) Jacoby tissue, and (5) peripheral glial mantle of Graefe. (B) 3D map of ONH with spectral domain OCT Heidelberg [superficial nerve fibre layer (SNFL); prelaminar region (PR); laminar region (LR); retrolaminar region (RLR)] ((A) modified with permission from Triviño et al. [29]).

This portion extends backwards and medially from the back of the eye to the optic canal in the sphenoid at the apex of the orbit. It is covered by three layers of meninges: the pia, the arachnoid and the dura mater [1, 2] (**Figure 9A**). The central retinal vessels must cross the subarachnoid space (between the pia and the arachnoid) and are therefore vulnerable, particularly the vein, in cases of raised intracranial pressure [2].

The intraorbital portion of the ON has a slight S-shaped bend, which allows a full range of ocular movement without stretching the nerve [1, 2]. As the ON approaches the orbital apex,

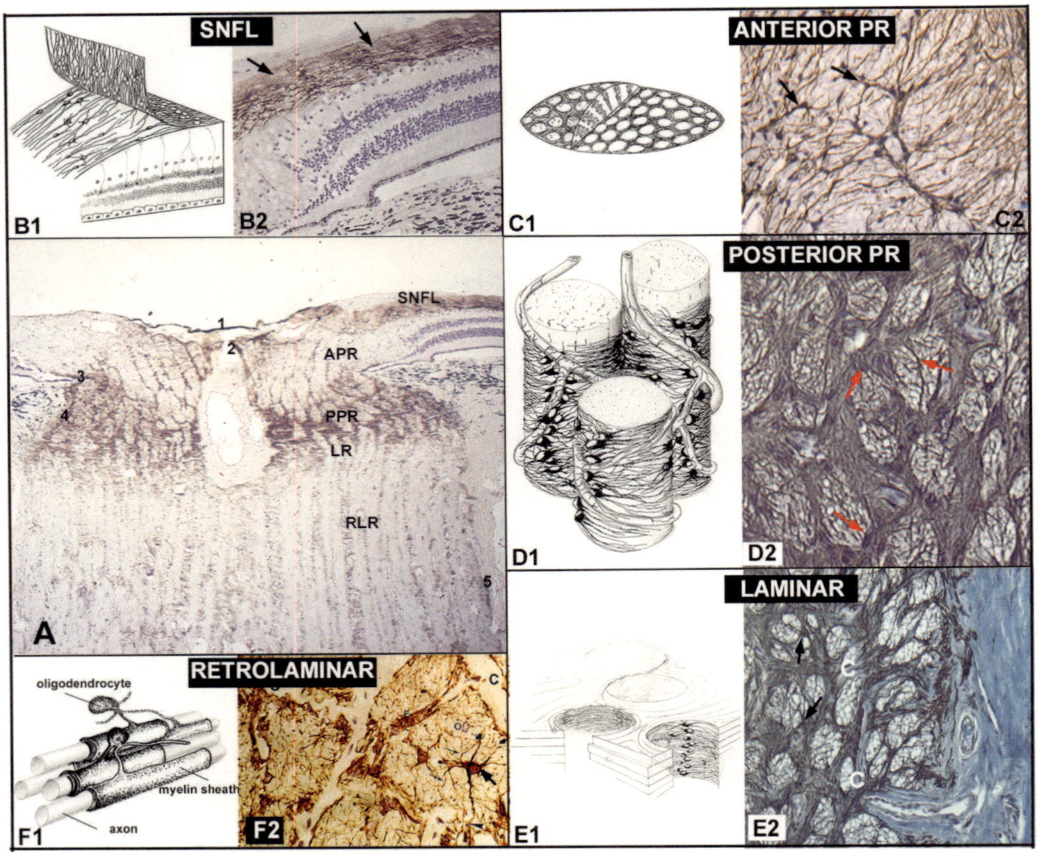

Figure 3. Morphology and distribution of astrocytes of the human optic nerve (O. N.). (A) Histological section of ON head. Superficial nerve fibre layer (SNFL), anterior prelaminar region (APR), posterior prelaminar region (PPR), laminar region (LR), and retrolaminar region (RLR). (1) Elschnig internal limiting membrane, (2) Kuhnt central meniscus, (3) Kuhnt intermediary tissue, (4) Jacoby tissue, and (5) peripheral glial mantle of Graefe. (B) Superficial nerve fibre layer: (B1) three-dimensional scheme and (B2) histological section. (C) Anterior prelaminar region: (C1) three-dimensional scheme and (C2) glioarchitecture. (D) Posterior prelaminar region: (D1) a three-dimensional diagram of the glial tubes and (D2) glioarchitecture. (E) Laminar region: (E1) three-dimensional scheme with pores covered with astroglia and (E2) histological section. (F) Retrolaminar region: (F1) scheme of myelin sheath forming by oligodendrocytes and (F2) histological section [astrocytes (arrows), collagen (C), oligodendrocytes (O), vessels (v)]. PAP immunohistochemistry: GFAP-PAP-haematoxylin (A, B2, F2) and GFAP Calleja's stain (C2, D2, E2) (B1,C1,C2,D1,F2,E1; modified with permission from Triviño et al. [29]).

it is surrounded by the tendinous annulus of Zinn, which has its origin in the rectus muscles [2, 4] (**Figure 1**).

- Intracanalicular (4–10 mm)

The intracanalicular portion of the ON passes through the optic canal, accompanied by the ophthalmic artery and the sympathetic nerves [2].

- Intracranial portion (10 mm)

The optic nerves leave the cranial end of the optic canal and pass medially, backwards and slightly upwards within the subarachnoid space of the middle cranial fossa [2]. They end by forming the optic chiasma in the floor of the third ventricle [1, 2].

The visual field (VF) can detect the alterations in nerve fibres [3]. The alterations of the different main bundles cause the following defects:

- In the papillomacular bundle (macular fibres that enter the temporal area of the disc): the central scotoma, the centrocecal scotoma and the paracentral scotoma
- In the arcuate nerve fibre bundle (fibres from the temporal retina to the disc that enters to disc in the superior and inferior poles): the arcuate Bjerrum's scotoma, Seidel's scotoma, the nasal step and the isolated scotoma within arcuate area
- In the nasal nerve fibre bundle (fibres that enter the nasal area of the disc in non-arcuate fashion, 'straight'): wedge-shaped temporal scotoma arising from the blind spot and does not necessarily respect the temporal horizontal meridian

The analysis of retinal axons using OCT allows us to detect axonal loss in vivo. The OCT technique and scanning laser polarimetry with variable corneal compensation (GDx, Carl Zeiss Meditec) are used to measure retinal nerve fibre layer (RNFL) thickness. The peripapillary RNFL has the advantage that the axons are unmyelinated, and any change is not confounded by demyelination as is the case of the optic nerve itself. Thinning of the peripapillary RNFL has been detected in patients with glaucoma, optic neuritis, multiple sclerosis, neuromyelitis optica, Alzheimer disease, Parkinson disease and other diseases. However, the patterns of change differ in some aspects.

1.3. The optic chiasma

It is situated at the junction of the anterior wall and the floor of the third ventricle [1], approximately 5–10 mm above the diaphragma sellae and the hypophysis cerebri [2]. Fifty-five percent of ON fibres cross in the chiasm [4]. This partial crossing of ON fibres is an essential requirement for binocular vision [2]. The fibres from the nasal hemiretina of each eye cross the midline to enter the contralateral optic tract after taking a short loop in the ipsilateral tract or into the contralateral optic nerve. Nerve fibres from the temporal hemiretina do not cross at the chiasma [2]. Macular fibres run posteriorly and centrally [3, 4]. Nasal fibres of the ipsilateral eye cross the chiasma and join the uncrossed temporal fibres of the contralateral eye [3]. Lower retina fibres lie laterally in the tracts and upper retinal fibres will lie medially.

Inferonasal retinal fibres cross into the chiasm anteriorly, approximately 4 mm into the contralateral ON, before running posteriorly forming 'Willebrand's knee' [3, 4].

The lesion of the nervous fibres at the level of chiasma, recorded by a VF, produces a bitemporal hemianopia due to the interruption of decussating nasal fibres [3]. When 'Willebrand's knee' is affected, it produces junctional scotoma [3, 4].

Using the OCT technique, diverse patterns of GCC loss in patients with chiasmal compression have been described. In addition, binasal GCC loss was typical and could be seen with minimal or no detectable VF loss. Moreover, thinning of the GCC may be detected before loss of the RNFL in some patients. After chiasmal decompression, the majority of patients showed an improvement in VF despite persistent GCC loss. Patients with less GCC loss before decompression had better postoperative VF.

1.4. The optic tracts

The optic tracts wind around the cerebral peduncles of the rostral midbrain, and they each divide into two roots. The first one is a large lateral root, which terminates posteriorly in the LGN and is related with a conscious visual sensation. The second one is a smaller medial root, which is connected both to the pretectal area and to the superior colliculus by the superior brachium and carries around 10% of tract fibres. This medial root functionally is not concerned with conscious vision [1, 2].

Lower retinal fibres and their projections lie in the lateral portion of the optic tract and terminate in the inferior striate cortex on the lower bank of the calcarine fissure. Upper retinal fibres project through the medial optic tract and ultimately terminate in the superior striate cortex [3].

The lateral root of the optic tract passes backwards, a little upwards, and terminates in the LGN, a part of the thalamus (a relay station for ascending sensory information). There is a 90° rotation (90° inward twist) of fibres from the nerves through the chiasm into the tracts (4) as it passes around the cerebral peduncles [2]. Macular fibres run centrally [1].

Damage to optic tract results in contralateral relative afferent pupillary defect (RAPD) because 55% of fibres cross [3, 4].

Optic tract lesion is an uncommon clinical entity. The primary characteristic is a homonymous VF defect that may be complete or incomplete. When the defect is incomplete, there is relative incongruity. When it is complete, there is an associated contralateral RAPD. Visual acuity and colour vision are preserved; unless there is bilateral involvement or anterior extension to involve the optic nerve or chiasm. When duration is enough, the contralateral fundus demonstrates a band or 'bow tie' atrophy of the disc and NFL.

The VF can detect alterations of the optic tract such as incongruous homonymous hemianopia (nerve fibres of corresponding points do not yet lie adjacent to one another). All retrochiasmatic lesions result in a contralateral homonymous hemianopia on the opposite side of the lesion. In general, the more posterior (towards the occipital cortex) the lesion is in postchiasmal visual pathways, the more likely the defects will be congruous [3].

1.5. Lateral geniculate nucleus (LGN)

Each LGN is distinguishable on the surface of the brain as an ovoid projection on the postero-inferior aspect of the thalamus, partly obscured by the overhanging temporal lobe [1, 2]. It consists of a body, head, spur and hilum. The hilum is continuous with the groove between the medial and lateral roots of the optic tract, which enters its anterior aspect. It lies at the anterior aspect of the pulvinar, which also partly surrounds it, particularly from above. Macular vision is subserved by the hilum and peripheral field by the medial and lateral horns [3].

The analysis by OCT shows that an uncrossed, temporal projection of the nerve fibre is affected in the eye ipsilateral to the damaged optic tract, resulting in preferential atrophy of the superior and inferior parts of the optic disc rim. In contrast, the crossed, nasal projection of the nerve fibres is damaged by the lesion in the contralateral eye, leading to the preferential atrophy of temporal and nasal parts of the optic disc rim, which is denoted as band atrophy.

In addition, Kanamori et al. [5] described reduced RNFL values in the contralateral eyes, the temporal and nasal (horizontal) by OCT. In contrast, the superior and inferior (vertical) RNFL were preferentially reduced compared to the horizontal RNFL, which are both located in the ipsilateral eyes. In the RNFL temporal-superior-nasal-inferior-temporal (TSNIT) profiles, a so-called double hump pattern, which represents thicker RNFL in the superior and inferior quadrants and thinner RNFL in the temporal and nasal quadrants, was preserved in the contralateral eyes but lost in the ipsilateral eyes. The analysis of the GCC using RTVue-OCT showed characteristic patterns of GCC thinning in both eyes, which is compatible with optic tract syndrome (OTS). The contralateral eyes showed an apparent GCC reduction from the nasal area to the fovea, whereas the ipsilateral eyes exhibited a significant GCC reduction from the temporal area to the fovea. GCC analysis provides information about the inner macular architecture. In this study, all cases exhibited marked changes in the GCC that were compatible with OTS but no changes in RNFL thickness. The RNFL in the superior and inferior parts of the optic nerve is composed of retinal nerve fibres originating from both temporal and nasal hemiretinal areas. In contrast, GCC temporal to the fovea in the temporal hemiretina comprise strictly retinal ganglion cell elements that reside within the corresponding areas. Such enrichment in retinal ganglion cell components, as well as stringent retinotopic segregation, may render the GCC superior to the circumpapillary retinal nerve fibre layer (cpRNFL) in the detection of homonymous hemianopic atrophy [5].

The LGN in which the great majority of the optic tract fibres terminate has a complex structure: it consists of six laminae or cell layers (numbered 1 to 6 beginning at the hilum), oriented in a dome-shaped mound similar to a stack of hats. Nerve fibres derived from the contralateral eye (crossed fibres from the nasal half of the retina) terminate on cell bodies in layers 1, 4 and 6. Those of the ipsilateral eye (uncrossed) terminate in layers 2, 3 and 5 [2, 4]. Thus, each LGN receives information from both retinae. Each retinal ganglion cell axon may terminate on up to six geniculate cells; however, these are located in one lamina. Fibres from the upper quadrants of peripheral retinae synapse on the medial aspect of the LGN and those of the lower quadrant on the lateral aspect. The macula projects to a disproportionately large central wedge of the LGN [2, 3]. Layers of LGN can also be categorized by neuronal size [4]:

- Magnocellular neurons (M cells): layers 1 and 2. These layers receive inputs from magnocellular RGCs. Magnocellular pathway is implicated in motion detection, stereoacuity and contrast sensitivity.
- Parvocellular neurons (P cells): layers 3 and 6. These layers receive inputs from parvocellular RGCs. Parvocellular pathway is implicated in fine spatial resolution and colour vision.
- Koniocellular neurons (K cells): These cells are located in interlaminar zones and superficial layers, receive inputs from both retinas and the superior colliculus and may modulate information.

The posterior aspect of the LGN is dome shaped, and it is from here that the geniculate cell axons form the optic radiation emerge [1, 2, 4]. The bulk of the LGN sends its fibres via the optic radiation to the visual cortex (area 17). The LGN has input from areas 17, 18 and 19, oculomotor centres and the reticular formation [2].

The alterations in the LGN, which are detected by the VF are [3]:

- Incongruous homonymous hemianopia
- Unique sector and sector-sparing defects due to a dual blood supply of LGN from anterior and posterior choroidal arteries

1.6. Postgeniculate pathway

1.6.1. Optic radiation

Optical radiation fibres show a certain order: the most anterior ones come from the lower part of the retina (upper VF) and the most posterior and dorsal ones from the upper part of the retina (lower VF) [1]. In the temporal lobe, fibres of the inferior retina are distributed as follows: the fibres of the inferotemporal part come from the ipsilateral eye, and the fibres of the inferior-nasal part are from the contralateral eye. They move anteriorly from the LGN and travel around ventricular system into the temporal lobe (Meyer's loop) [3, 4]. Inferior macular fibres do not cross as far anteriorly in the temporal lobe [3]. In the parietal lobe, fibres of the superior retina are distributed as follows: the superotemporal fibres come from the ipsilateral eye and the superonasal from the contralateral eye. They travel superiorly in the optic radiation, in white matter from the parietal cortex to the occipital lobe [3, 4]. Macular fibres travel more centrally [4].

The alterations of this pathway detected by VF are:

- Anterior temporal lobe lesions produce midperipheral and peripheral contralateral homonymous superior quadrantanopia ('pie in the sky' field defect); more extensive temporal lobe lesions may cause defects that extend to the inferior quadrants but 'denser' superiorly [3].
- Parietal lobe lesions tend to affect superior fibres first, resulting in contralateral inferior homonymous quadrantanopia or a homonymous hemianopia 'denser' inferiorly [3].
- The injury of a complete optic tract interrupts the fibres coming from the temporal half of one retina and of the nasal half the other, causing blindness in the right or left halves of both retinas. Whether the right or the left band is affected, it produces a homonymous hemianopia on the side contralateral to the affected band 1.

1.6.2. Primary visual cortex or Brodmann area 17

The central (30°) visual field occupies a disproportionately large area (68–83%) of the visual cortex [3]. The vertical meridians are represented along the border of the calcarine lips, while the horizontal meridian follows the contour of the base of the calcarine fissure [3].

Main defect types observed by the analysis of VF are the central homonymous hemianopia with or without macular sparing depending on the location of the lesion [3].

Using the OCT technique, it has been described that acquired unilateral damage to the occipital lobe resulting in homonymous hemianopia leads to nerve fibre layer thinning. Thinning of the GCL on the lesion's projecting sector of the macula has been described in lesions in the posterior visual pathway with a strong correlation between the corresponding macular segment of the GCL and the VF. In addition, the finding of sector macular GCL atrophy proves retrograde trans-synaptic degeneration of neurons in the visual pathway in cases without other ophthalmic or neurological diseases. It has been proposed that this is probably because at the macula, the bodies of the neurons are more numerous and topographically organized to correspond to the VF. In contrast, the anatomical distribution of fibres in the peripapillary RNFL is more complex, making a correlation with the visual field more difficult to establish. Another important element is the absence of blood vessels or other structures that may interfere with the OCT image acquisition. It is noteworthy that cases with macular sparing hemi- and quadrantanopia also showed macular GCL atrophy away from the fovea. It is perhaps explained the representation of a 15–20u of visual field in the area scanned by the OCT instrument used and the absence of ganglion cells on the fovea.

2. Microscopic anatomy and function of the optic nerve

The components of the optic nerve are:

- The axons of the RGCs
- Glial cells: astrocytes, oligodendrocytes and microglia
- The connective tissue: which constitutes the lamina cribrosa and the septa that fasciculate the optic nerve
- Blood vessels, derived from both the central retinal artery (CRA) system and the ciliary system

The intraocular nerve head can be divided into four parts (**Figure 2**):

- The superficial nerve fibre layer (**Figures 3A**, **B1** and **B2**)
- The prelaminar region (**Figures 3A**, **C1**, **C2**, **D1** and **D2**)
- The laminar region (**Figures 3A**, **E1** and **E2**)
- The retrolaminar region (which corresponds to the anterior portion of the intraorbital region) (**Figures 3A**, **F1** and **F2**)

The basic organization of the optic nerve head is similar in all regions. The axons of the RGCs form beams of several thousand axons each, which are surrounded by different tissues; the latter, however, are those that will vary in the different areas of the nerve.

2.1. Superficial nerve fibre layer

In the retina, the axons of the RGCs will converge towards the optic disc following a fairly straight trajectory, thus constituting the superficial nerve fibre layer (**Figures 3B1** and **B2**).

This layer is constituted by axonal bundles that are formed by the gathering of rows of axons that converge on their way to the optic disc. Therefore, an axonal bundle that reaches the optic nerve head will contain axons from RGCs, the location of which varies from the peripheral retina to the vicinity of the head of the optic nerve [6]. In addition, another characteristic of the axons of this region is where they are unmyelinated because there are no oligodendrocytes. The majority of glial type of this layer is made up of astrocytes (**Figure 3B1** and **B2**) [7].

The axons of the RGCs follow an established pattern. In addition, the presence of fovea in the human retina will affect the arrangement of the axons in this layer in such a way that the axons of the RGCs on the nasal side, both superior and inferior, are not affected by the fovea and go directly to the optic disc. The same thing happens with the RGCs of the nasal temporal retina to the fovea, the axons of which form the papillomacular bundle on their way to the optic disc [6]. However, the RGCs temporal to the fovea cannot go through this area to join the papillomacular bundle. Therefore, they surround the fovea forming arcs above and below it, as they go towards the optic disc (arcuate bundles). Temporal to the fovea, there is a dividing line (the horizontal raphe) which separates the RGCs, whose axons are going to pass over the fovea, from the RGCs, and whose axons are going below this line [6, 8–10].

With respect to the organization of the axons in the thickness of this layer, different theories have been postulated. Some propose that the axons of the RGCs located more peripherally are arranged closer to the GCL, while the axons closest to the optic nerve head go through the superficial NFL perpendicularly so as to arrange themselves close to the vitreous surface. Thus, the axons coming from the periphery, which are close to the GCL, rotate 90° in the margin of the optic disc, whereas the axons of the more central RGCs go close to the vitreous surface and rotate close to the centre of the optic nerve head [11, 12]. However, other studies defend that the peripheral RGCs have the most superficial axons, while the most central ones have their axons close to the GCL. Therefore, at the optic nerve head, the most peripheral axons that run close to the vitreous surface rotate 90° in the most peripheral part of the optic nerve, while the central axons rotate in the centre of the optic disc [13].

At present, it is believed that the organization of the superficial NFL in the vitreous-scleral thickness is not related to the axonal eccentricity but that the axons coming from CGRs of different areas are mixed in a wedge extending from the periphery to the centre of the optic nerve. As a result, the axons in this region would not be predetermined to establish a retinotopic order [14, 15].

With the recent advances in imaging technology using a spectral-domain, optical coherence tomography (SDOCt9), in particular the enhanced depth imaging (EDI) technique of SD OCT, quantitative assessment of the superficial NFL thickness is possible. Observations in the distribution of peripapillary choroid show that the inferior region of the optic nerve is the thickest in comparison with the other regions [16–19]. Some authors postulate the theory that both the vascular watershed zone and the embryogenic location of the optic fissure closure may be responsible [20]. One of the known reasons for the vulnerability of the lower region is that of the lamina cribrosa in the lower pole has large pores and thinner connective tissue and glial support for the retinal ganglion cell axons to pass [21–23]. Another speculation could be that the thinnest peripapillary choroid in the lower quadrant, which represents an area of lower blood supply, may predispose the lower region of the optic nerve to glaucomatous ischemic damage [24].

2.1.1. *Axoplasmic flow*

For axons grow and maintain their structural integrity, it is necessary that there be an intra-axonal particle movement known as the axoplasmic flow. This flow is bidirectional in such a way that the molecules are transported from the soma to the axon and from axon to the synapse or from the synapse to the soma [25]. This soma-synapsis communication is important in the case of neurons with long axons such as RGCs in which the axon has to travel a long way to reach the LGN [26]. Although most of the cytoplasmic organelles involved in protein synthesis are found in the neuronal soma, axons have a certain capacity for synthesis. The transported molecules vary substantially from filamentous components of the axon and proteins to mitochondria, secretory granules or multivesicular bodies [27].

The axoplasmic flow can be divided into [25, 26]:

a. Orthograde or antegrade: the direction of movement is from soma to synapse. It is involved in axonal growth and maintenance of the synapse. Three subtypes can be differentiated:

  1. Fast: the driving speed ranges between 100 and 500 mm/day. Mainly, membranous cell structures, neurotransmitters, hydrolases and soluble materials of low molecular weight are transported.
  2. Intermediate: the driving speed oscillates between 5 and 50 mm/day.
  3. Slow: the driving speed oscillates between 0.5 and 3 mm/day. It constitutes 80% of the total protein flow and is responsible for the transport of soluble proteins that form the structure of the axon. This is how structural elements of1 the axon, soluble enzymes and proteins travel.

b. Retrograde: it goes from the axon to the cell body. It carries a driving speed of about 200 mm/day. This flow is responsible for transporting the cellular detritus resulting from axon metabolism, aged organelles, fragments and membrane proteins towards the lysosomal compartment of the neuronal soma for its degradation and reuse or its definitive disablement. Furthermore, the retrograde flow serves to inform the cell body of the state of the axon terminal.

When axoplasmic flow is blocked, axons undergo a series of damage that leads to oedema, necrosis and optic atrophy. This has been demonstrated experimentally after the induction of different pathologies such as glaucoma, ischemic optic neuropathy or papilledema due to intracranial hypertension [28] (**Figure 4A**).

2.1.2. *Astroglia*

Other main constituents of the optic nerve are the astrocytes. In the superficial NFL, astrocytes have a thin cell body and their processes run parallel to the RGC axons (**Figure 3B1** and **B2**) [29, 30]. Under normal conditions, astrocytes establish contact with retinal neurons, providing stability to neural tissue [31]. Physiological studies have highlighted the important functions performed by these cells in the optic nerve and other parts of the CNS. Thus, they

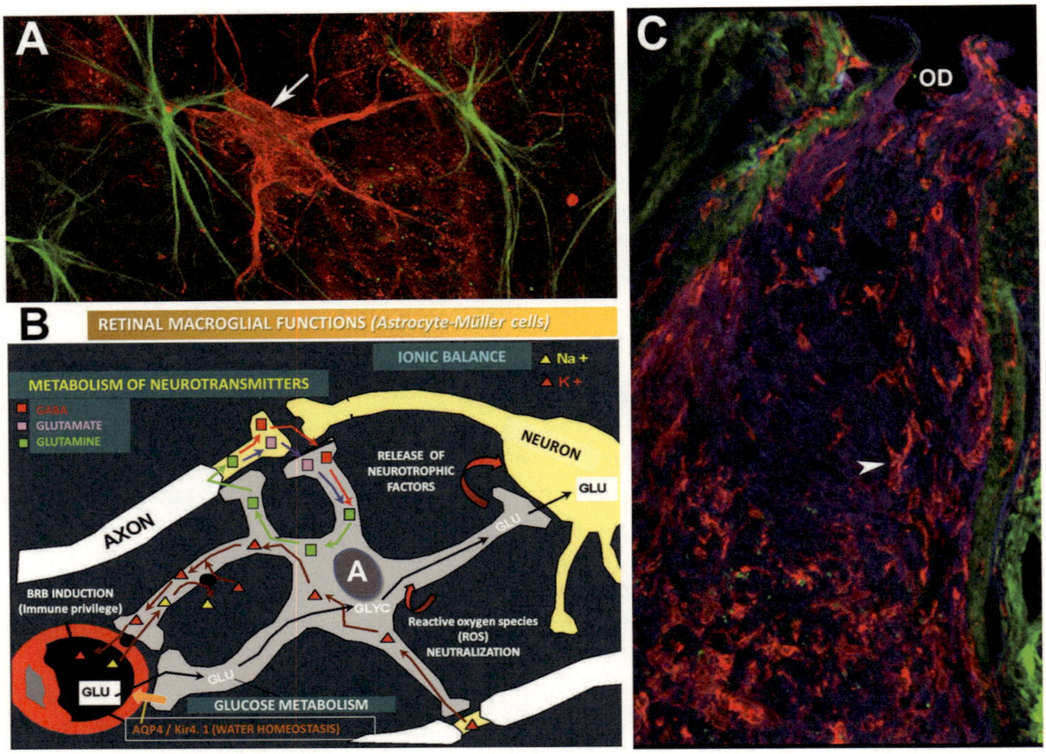

Figure 4. (A) Blockade of the axoplasmic flow. NF-200 (+) retinal ganglion cell in red (arrow), with an accumulation of neurofilaments in its cytoplasm by blocking its axoplasmic flow, in an experimental glaucoma model. In green, astrocytes GFAP(+). Retinal whole-mount immunofluorescence. (B) Scheme of the astroglia functions. (C) Microglia in the optic nerve. Iba-1+ ramified microglia (arrowhead) were observed. Immunofluorescence of the optic nerve section. Iba1+ in red and GFAP+ in blue. Optic disc (OD) ((A) modified with permission from Gallego et al. [73], (B) modified with permission from Ramírez et al. [181]).

are responsible for the storage of glycogen by providing glucose to the neurons. They regulate extracellular potassium levels. They play an important role in the regulation and metabolism of neurotransmitters such as GABA. They help in the elimination of retinal CO2. They contribute to the maintenance of water homeostasis in the retina [27, 32–36]. Moreover, they are the inducers of the blood-retinal barrier properties (**Figure 4B**) [37]. At the level of the optic nerve, astrocytes are responsible for the fasciculation of axons [38, 39].

On the superficial NFL, there is a second morphological type of astrocytes, with a thick cell body and short processes. Its function is to separate and protect the optic nerve axons from the surrounding tissues, since they make up a series of glial limiting membranes:

a. Elschnig's limiting membrane (**Figures 3A** and **5A1**), which isolates the ganglion cell axons from the vitreous surface

b. The Kuhnt central meniscus (**Figures 3A** and **5A1**). Elschnig's limiting membrane is quite thick in the physiologic cup and constitutes this central meniscus. This is in continuity with glial tissue surrounding the adventitia of the central vessels (CRA and central retinal vein) [29, 30].

The main role attributed to these limiting glial membranes is to induce the blood-optic nerve barrier, which prevents the passage of molecules between the optic nerve and the adjacent tissues, which in this case is the vitreous body and the optic nerve vessels [30, 40].

2.1.3. Vascularization

The vessels that nourish the superficial NFL are dependent on the main retinal arterioles. The capillaries of this area continue along with the retinal peripapillary capillaries and the radial peripapillary capillary (RPC) network. Sometimes, there may be a vascular contribution from the prelaminar region by vessels derived from the ciliary system (**Figure 5A2**) [41–44].

The RPCs in the human retina were first described by Michaelson [45] as a unique plexus in their distribution to the posterior pole and seemed to be oriented parallel to the RNFL axons. Henkind [46] noted that the RPCs are the most superficial layer of capillaries lying in the inner part of the RNFL, and they run along the paths of the major superotemporal and inferotemporal vessels up to 4 to 5 mm from the optic nerve head (ONH). The RPCs have a distinctive and easily recognizable pattern of parallel, long, uniform-diameter vessels that remain within RNFL layers [47]. Henkind reported [46, 48] that in macaques and humans, RCPs are most prominent in the Bjerrum's region and are absent in the central macular region. RPCs have a long linear trajectory oriented parallel to the adjacent capillaries and radiate anteriorly from the ONH, forming only a few anastomoses with adjacent vessels [49]. In this region, retinal venous pulsations occur spontaneously in up to 95% of normal human eyes [50]. Some authors have identified that some major factors inherent to the retinal vein, as well as their relationship to surrounding optic disc structures, may influence some characteristics such as venous diameter, the presence of arteriovenous crossings and tissue depth, which affect sites of venous pulsation. Changes in venous compliance may affect venous pulsations in various retinal vascular diseases like diabetic retinopathy and venous occlusive disease, as well as glaucoma [51].

2.2. The prelaminar region

In the prelaminar region (PR), the axons of the CGRs change their trajectory, curving 90° to move towards the optic chiasm. This zone is also known as the choroidal region of the lamina cribrosa (**Figures 2** and **3A**) [41–44, 52].

In this region, two zones can be differentiated depending on the organization, arrangement, density and morphology of the astrocytes, as well as the way these cells fasciculate the axons. These two areas are the anterior PR (**Figures 3C1** and **C2**) and the posterior PR (**Figure 3D1** and **D2**) [29, 30].

2.2.1. Anterior prelaminar region

In the anterior PR, astrocytes are characterized by a stellate morphology with a thin cell body. Its disposition is closely related to the distribution pattern presented by the vascular system (**Figures 3C1**, **C2** and **5B2**) [30]. The vessels of this region derive from the ciliary system from the prechoriocapillary peripapillary choroid and can sometimes contribute to centripetal vessels from the circle of Zinn-Haller (**Figure 5B1** and **B2**) [8, 41, 44, 53, 54].

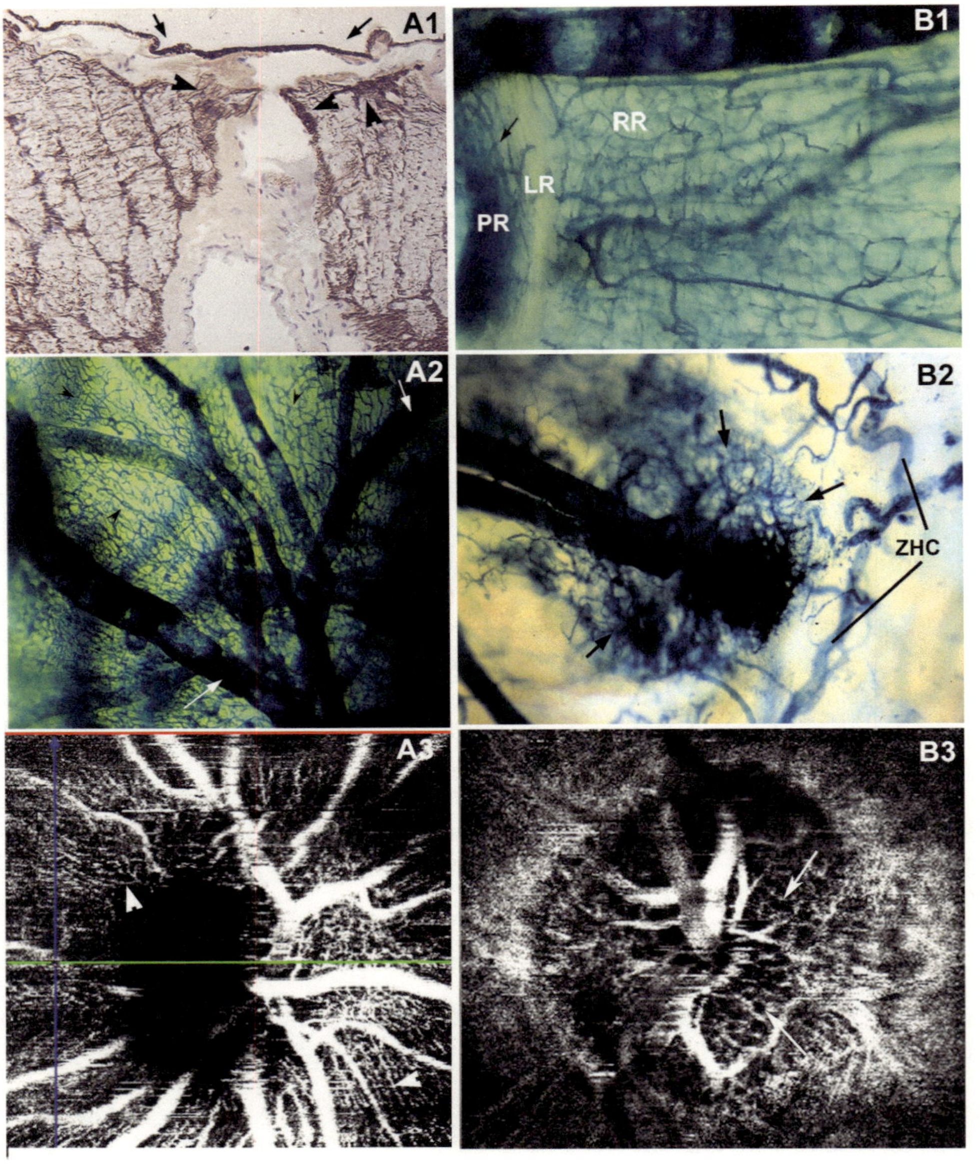

Figure 5. (A) Superficial nerve fibre layer (SNFL): (A1) Elschnig internal limiting membrane (arrows) and Kuhnt central meniscus (arrowhead). (A2) vascularization of the SNFL. Main branches of the artery and central vein of the retina (arrow) and capillary vascular bed (arrowhead). (A3) radial peripapillary capillaries (arrowhead). (B) Prelaminar region of the optic nerve head (ONH). (B1) lateral view of the vascularization of the ONH. Prelaminar region (PR), laminar region (LR), and retrolaminar region (RR). (B2, B3) vascularization of the prelaminar region (arrows). Zinn-Haller circle (CZH) ((A1) immunohistochemistry GFAP-PAP-Ünna Tanzer; (A2, B1, B2) diaphanization technique and vascular filling with polymers. (A3, B3) SD angio OCT Heidelberg).

Thin-bodied stellate astrocytes are the predominant cells in this region. Their cell bodies are basically positioned over blood vessels and emit primary processes in the direction of the vessel walls to make up an astroglial net that form a basket-like structure through whose compartments the axons pass (**Figure 3A**, **C1** and **C2**) [30]. The layout of the astrocytes at this level reflects their supporting and protective function with respect to the myelinated fibres at the place in which they bend 90 degrees. These astrocytes may also have an important mechanical role as they could impede possible squeezing and rubbing among the nerve axons. This structure is relatively elastic if it is compared with the rigidity of the scleral lamina cribrosa. This elasticity may ameliorate or prevent irreparable nerve fibre damage when the disc swells from papilledema or neuritis [30].

2.2.2. Posterior prelaminar region

The basket-like structure of the anterior PR is substituted in the posterior PR by glial tubes (**Figure 3A**, **D1** and **D2**). The astrocytes of this region have thick bodies and form glial tubes through which the axons run. The blood vessels will be arranged between the thick glia partitions that make up the walls of these tubes (**Figures 3D1** and **D2**) [29, 30]. As in the anterior PR, these cells make up a structure through which the vessels that penetrate the nerve from the adjacent choroid run and form a pericapillary net with an irregular morphology. These glial tubes may have the mechanical function of resisting the pressures that originate at this level when the eyes move. The tubes surround the nerve fibres like a sheath. A number of data seem to support this glial function in the posterior PR: first, the abundance of GFAP supplies the astroglial processes with some tensile strength [55]. Thus, the richness of GFA protein observed in electron microscopy in the astroglial cells of this area would be providing a certain tensional force to the astroglial extensions [29, 30, 52, 56], and second, the presence of desmosomes [57] and gap junctions [58] supports this possibility. Both types of junction may have an important role in maintaining the astroglial net through which the axons pass, since even under high osmotic pressures the gap junctions remain intact. In addition, these glial tubes are organizing the axonal bundles preparing them for entry into the laminar region (LR), which is clearly seen in the transition zone between both regions where it can be seen how the glial tubes are perfectly matched with the cribrosa pores [29, 30, 41].

2.2.3. Limiting membranes

In the prelaminar region, we find two other glial limiting membranes: the Kuhnt intermediary tissue, which separates the optic nerve from the retina, and it continues subsequently with the border tissue of Jacoby, which isolates the optic nerve from the surrounding choroidal tissue (**Figures 2A**, **3A** and **5A1**) [29, 41, 57, 59, 60].

Both limiting membranes are formed by thick cell body astrocytes that are arranged in densely packed 4–5 layers forming a separation barrier between the optic nerve, the retina and the choroid [29]. The barrier function is supported by the existence of tight junctions between the astrocytes of the Kuhnt intermediary tissue and the retinal pigment epithelium cells as well as the presence of desmosomes between the astrocytes and the outer limiting membrane [60]. This barrier function could explain the large number of myelin fragments and dense bodies, which are phagocytosed and degraded by the astrocytes that form these glial limiting membranes [29, 59].

Another function fundamentally attributed to the Kuhnt and Jacoby tissues is that they act as bearings that cushion the frictions that take place in the small displacements of the optic nerve during the movements of the eyeball. In this way, the suffering of the nerve fibres, which enter the nerve in the peripheral areas, is avoided. This can be corroborated by the parallel disposition of the astroglial processes, which are connected to each other by numerous desmosome and tight junctions. Furthermore, the large number of intermediate filaments existing in these astroglial processes would provide them a certain rigidity and tensile force [29, 30, 52, 55, 57, 60].

2.2.4. *Microglia*

In the PR, as in the rest of the ON, in addition to the astrocytes, we find microglial cells. Microglia is a subtype of glia of the central nervous system that is activated in response to neuronal damage [61, 62]. In the normal tissue, these cells are quiescent and have a branched shape with a small nucleus and a cell body with several processes (**Figure 4C**).

At the ONH, quiescent microglial cells (which are HLA-DR, CD45 and Iba-1+) are located on the walls of the large vessels, surrounding the capillaries in the glial columns of the PR and the cribriform pores of the LR. In the case of moderate or severe damage in the ONH, the microglia are activated [63–65], forming accumulations of amoeboid microglia in the lamina cribrosa and surrounding blood vessels [66, 67].

2.3. The laminar region

The lamina cribrosa (LC) forms a band of dense, compact connective tissue across the scleral foramen. Its sieve-like arrangement (the lamina cribrosa) transmits the axon bundles of the nerve and central retinal vessels through a series of round or oval apertures (pores) embraced by strong trabeculae [68]. In normal eyes, the number of pores that form the LC is among 550–650. Histologically, it has been estimated that the diameter of the pores varies between 10 and 100 μm and that it decreases towards the posterior part of the LC (**Figure 6A**) [69, 70]. The bulk of the LC is made up of a series of dense connective sheets (**Figures 3E1** and **E2**). The LC blend peripherally with the sclera and alternate with a series of glial sheets in a lamellar fashion. LC plates are composed of elastin; collagen types I, III, IV and VI; laminin; and heparan sulphate proteoglycan [52, 73–75]. The collagens and the elastic fibres act as shock absorbers of the tension that supports this area of the optic nerve. Proteoglycans play an important role in the biomechanical properties of tissues, in such a way that, by occupying an extensive volume in relation to their molecular weights, they can be compressed before a load and expanded when it disappears. As in the optic nerve, there is a gradient of hydrostatic pressure from the disc to the retrolaminar region [76]; the properties of these molecules are important to soften the pressure gradient [66].

Using trypsin digestion and scanning electron microscopy, it is possible to appreciate the structure of the LC plates. There are regional variations in the form of the LC plates. Therefore, the superior and inferior quadrants of the laminar sheets are thinner and sparser, resulting in the formation of larger pores than in the nasal and temporal quadrants (**Figures 6B** and **C**) [21, 69].

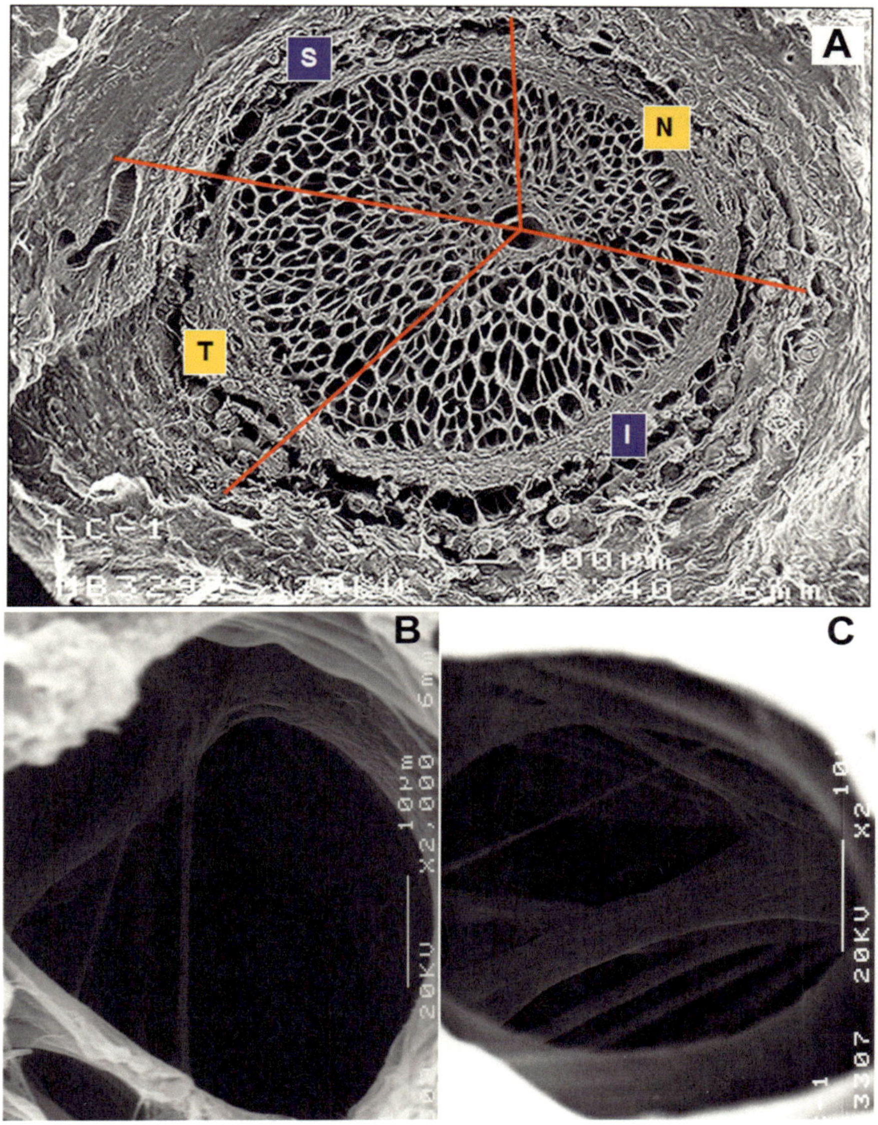

Figure 6. (A) Laminar region of the optic nerve head: Superior (S), nasal (N), inferior (I) and temporal (T) sectors. (B, C) detail of the cribriform pores: (B) nasal cribriform pore and (C) inferotemporal cribriform pore. (A–C) scanning electron microscopy with nervous tissue digestion by trypsin. (A: modified with permission from Ramírez et al. [181]).

There are two cellular types coating the LC plates: the LC cells and astrocytes (**Figure 3E2**). LC cells have been described as large, flat, broad and polygonal GFAP (−) alpha-smooth muscle actin (alpha-SMA)+ cells that possess multiple cell processes [71]. However, they take on a more oval shape in situ [72]. Although LC cells reside within the LC, astrocytes GFAP (+) are located in the plate openings alongside axon bundles as they transverse multiple plates [66, 71]. Ultrastructural evaluations show that LC cells are elongated with abundant cytoplasmic actin microfilaments and organelles, such as an active rough endoplasmic reticulum, a well-developed Golgi apparatus and a dense band of heterochromatin along the nuclear membrane [77]. LC cells produce an increased expression of extracellular matrix (ECM) proteins if exposed to mechanical stimulation [78]. LC cells are now recognized as a major site of RGC damage in primary open-angle glaucoma. Cells within the LC have profound effects on the ECM environment and RGC survival. Autocrine or paracrine signaling of growth factors between cells of the LC may play a role in maintaining a homeostatic mechanism within the human LC [79].

Ganglion cell axons go through the pores of the LC. Most of the nerve fibres that pass through the lamina cribrosa take a direct course. However, between 8 and 12% of the fibres can be diverted to pass through the cribriform pores in the central and peripheral areas of the disc. Consequently, these axons could be more vulnerable to alterations of the LC [76].

It has been proven that there are significant correlations between the area, convexity and aspect ratio of a pore and the level of biomechanical insult to the neural tissues within the pore. The relationship between pore shape and neural tissue insult was observed for undeformed configurations. When deformed by intraocular pressure (IOP)-induced hoop stress, the pores became larger and more convex possibly reducing the risk for further insult [80].

It has been observed that damage to the neuroretinal rim in moderate glaucoma occurred mainly in the inferotemporal [81] and superotemporal regions [82], while the remaining portions of the neuroretinal ring in advanced glaucoma were found in the nasal region [82]. Quigley and Addicks [83] performed a histological evaluation of optic nerve axons at the LC and found that axon loss occurred in all regions but was greater in the superior and inferior regions of the LC. Furthermore, the pattern of axon loss corresponded to regional differences in the structure of the LC, which contained larger pores and thinner beams in the superior and inferior regions [22].

2.3.1. Glioarchitecture of the laminar region

With respect to the glioarchitecture of this region, there is a marked decrease in glial tissue, which only covers the internal face of LC plates (**Figures 3E1** and **E2**). The astrocytes have a thick cell body similar to those of the posterior PR but form a single layer that covers the inner wall of the LC pores (**Figures 3E1** and **E2**). The function of these cells is to provide functional support to axons and synthesize macromolecules of the extracellular matrix, which is also responsible for supporting the shearing and stretching forces generated by the displacement of the LC by the action of IOP [29, 30, 41, 84].

The core of the cribriform plates is separated from the astrocytes by a continuous and well-defined layer of type IV collagen, laminin and heparan sulphate proteoglycan (**Figures 3E1** and **E2**). These macromolecules form part of the basement membrane of astrocytes and contribute to form a network of filamentous material. This basement membrane fulfils a structural function by providing a flexible substrate for cell attachment. In addition, laminin plays an important role in the regulation of cell differentiation and proliferation of neural tissues [66, 76].

Cells are anchored to the basement membrane by membrane glycoproteins with adherent properties, having identified in the optic nerve by one of the main types of adhesion molecules, integrins [66].

Regarding their embryonic origin, the glial elements of the ONH are derived from ectodermal cells, but the mesenchymal cells of neural crest account for the development of the LC tissue and cells [77].

It is possible that LC cells are astrocyte precursors or develop into astrocytes because there is a large GFAP subpopulation of astrocytes existing in the brain [85, 86]. Thus, LC cells may be a subset of GFAP astrocytes but are different from the normal ONH astrocytes because of their different morphologies and immunostaining properties [72].

2.3.2. *Vascularization of the laminar region*

The LC is supplied by centripetal branches arising directly from the short posterior ciliary arteries or from the intrascleral circle of Zinn and Haller (**Figures 7A** and **8A**).

The posterior ciliary arteries (PCAs) originate from the ophthalmic artery and enter the ocular globe laterally, medially or superiorly to the optic nerve, which is why they are denominated lateral, medial or superior PCAs. The number of these vessels shows a marked interindividual variation (between one and five) [87] although the most frequent situation is the existence of two to three PCAs (**Figure 7A**) [88, 89].

In the case that there are only two PCAs (medial and lateral), these vessels irrigate the nasal and temporal portion of the choroid, respectively, finding a watershed zone that is the border between the territories of distribution of adjacent end arteries. Since the PCA circulation is the main source of blood supply to the optic nerve head, the location of the watershed zone between the PCAs is crucial in ischemic disorders of the ONH. This watershed usually runs vertically somewhere in the area between the fovea and the peripapillary nasal choroid (**Figure 7B**) [90–92]. On the other hand, if there are three or more PCAs, the watershed is usually Y-shaped, and it is located in a part of the optic disc. However, there may be different combinations of shapes in the watershed zones when there are more than two PCAs, depending on whether the area supplied by each PCA is a quadrant or only one sector. Thus, when the entire optic disc lies in the centre of a watershed zone, that disc is particularly vulnerable to ischemia [88, 89, 91, 93].

The ACPs are subdivided into several branches before perforating the sclera, which surrounds the optic disc. They are two long posterior ciliary arteries (LPCAs) and 15–20 short posterior ciliary arteries (SPCA) (**Figure 7A**) [94–96]. According to their scleral penetration, the SPCAs can be subdivided into para-optic SPCAs (closer to the optic disc) and distal SPCAs (**Figure 7A**) [97, 98].

In histological sections, SPCAs and LPCAs are characterized because they have the typical structure of small arteries with an endothelium and internal elastic lamina in the tunica intima, two smooth muscular layers in the tunica media and an adventitia constituted by circularly oriented collagen. The arterioles derived from these arteries present an endothelium covered with a basement membrane, a discontinuous muscular layer and a continuous collagen adventitia [9, 99–101].

Overall, two para-optic SPCAs penetrate and surround the optic disc constituting the Zinn-Haller arterial circle, which provides blood flow to the circumpapillary choroid and the prelaminar and

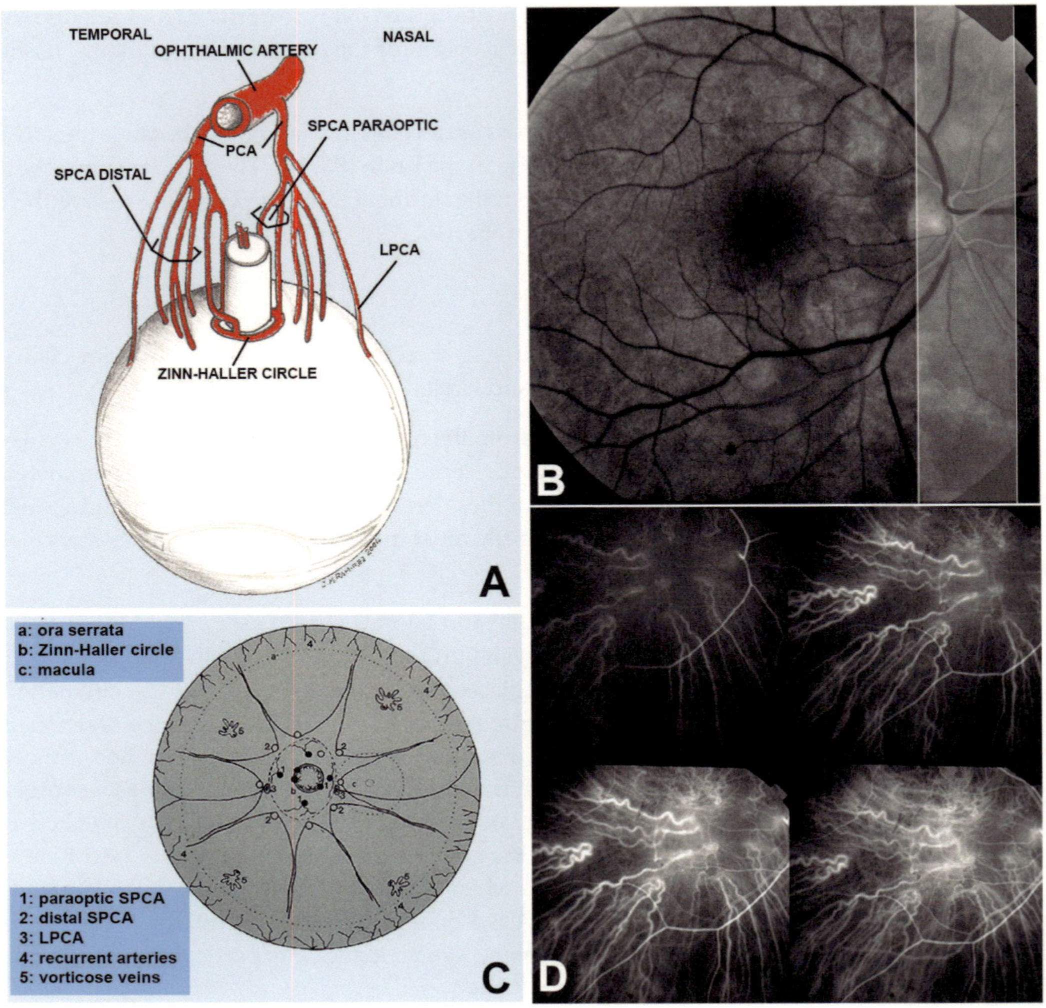

Figure 7. Ciliary system vascularization. (A) Three-dimensional scheme of the ciliary artery entrance in the eyeball. (B) Fluorescein angiography showing the watershed between the territories of the PCA (space between lines). (C) Scheme of the distribution of the branches of the PSCA in the human choroid. (D) Indocyanine green angiography of the sectoral division of the PSCAs that form triangular areas and the watershed zones between these branches [posterior ciliary arteries (PCA), short posterior ciliary arteries (SPCA), long posterior ciliary arteries (LPCA)].

laminar regions of the ONH, through capillaries originating directly from the Zinn-Haller circle (**Figures 5B2**, **7A** and **8A**). The rest of the SPCAs, both para-optic and distal, once in the choroidal vascular layer, divide sectorially forming triangular areas towards the four regions of the eyeball. These arterial ramifications (which generate the choroidal arteries) first are dichotomous, forming acute angles. The posterior ramifications can do so from acute angles to angles of 180°, carrying during its travel an undulating trajectory (**Figures 7C** and **D**) [94–96, 102].

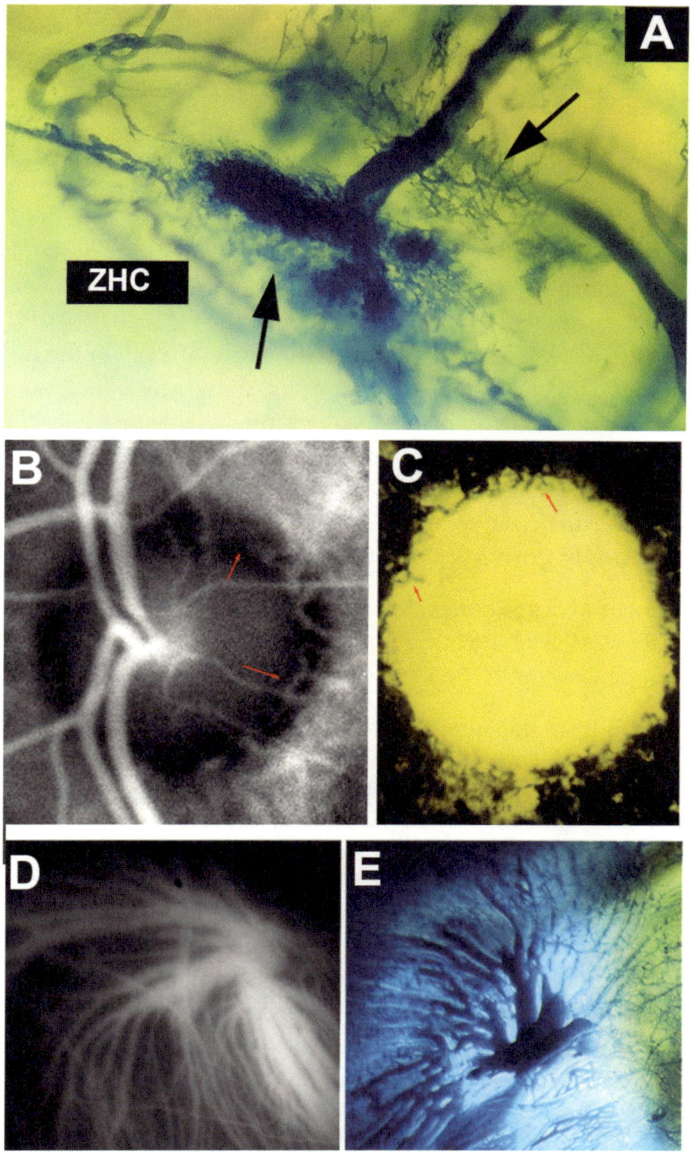

Figure 8. Ciliary system vascularization. (A) Zinn-Haller arterial circle (ZHC) (arrows) dependent on two short posterior ciliary arteries. (B, C) vascular branches of choroidal peripapillary precoriocapilar. Centripetal vessels (arrows). (D, E) Vorticose veins. (A, C, E) Diaphanization technique and vascular filling with polymers. (B) Fluorescein angiography. (D) Angiography with indocyanine green.

The macular region is irrigated by distal branches of the SPCAs, without observing, contrary to what was postulated by some authors (90–92) in any specific vessel for this region [96, 103–106]. The macular region is irrigated by a dense network of distal branches of SPCAs

[94]. Furthermore, this region corresponds to the area of the choroids, which presents a higher blood perfusion pressure and higher blood flow [107, 108].

The peripapillary region is mainly irrigated by para-optic branches of SPCAs and some branches from the Zinn-Haller arterial circle. This circle emits branches not only for prechoriocapillary peripapillary choroid but also for the PR and LR of the ONH (**Figure 8B** and **C**) [48, 96, 108–110].

Posterior ciliary arteries are end arteries. However, they are not completely so in the functional sense, because choroidal vascular occlusions frequently recover over a matter of days [90, 106, 111, 112]. There are watershed zones between the various PCAs (**Figure 7B** and **D**). The significance of the watershed zone is that in the event of a fall in the perfusion pressure in the vascular bed of one or more of the end arteries, the watershed zone, being an area of comparatively poor vascularity, is most vulnerable to ischemia [90, 111]. The existence of these watershed zones has been demonstrated between PCAs [90], SPCAs [106], SPCAs and LPCAs [113], anterior ciliary arteries and PCAs [112, 114], lobule of choriocapillaris [112, 115, 116] and the vorticose veins [112]. Moreover, its location on the macular region and the ONH could imply greater vulnerability of these areas to chronic ischemia [91].

The arterial and venous systems of the choroid are not parallel as they are in most systems of the body. Most of the vessels of the outermost choroid are mainly veins with the exception of those close to the optic disc and those located under the macula [117].

The veins collect blood from the anterior uvea, from the equator and from the posterior pole, to drain the entire choroid via vorticose veins. The choroidal venules and veins are larger than the arteries and maintain a rectilinear path, joining at many acute angles before ending in the vorticose veins [9, 99, 117].

Normally, there are four vorticose veins, two nasal (superior and inferior) and two temporal (superior and inferior) [118], although this number can vary between three and six. These veins are located equatorially (one for each quadrant) and form a bottle shape receptacle before its scleral perforation, which is accordingly constituted by the meeting of two to four ampulliform dilatations (**Figure 8D** and **E**) [97, 119]. Histologically, the veins present an endothelium (with its basement membrane), an irregular muscular layer and a fine collagen adventitia. Venules are broadly similar but have no muscle layer [99].

Classically, it has been described that each vorticose vein and its tributaries drained a quadrant of the choroid with little or no overlap between the other adjacent drainage quadrants. A boundary or edge (watershed) exists between these territories [120]. These limiting zones are arranged in the form of a cross, which crosses near the posterior pole, with the horizontal arm passing through the optic disc and the macula and the vertical arm between the optic disc and the macula [120]. Therefore, the temporal quadrant on the horizontal plane would be drained by the superior temporal vorticose vein, whereas the inferior temporal quadrant would be drained by the inferior temporal vorticose vein. According to this interpretation, these watershed areas would be regions that could be more affected by venous occlusions.

http://dx.doi.org/10.5772/intechopen.79827

However, this interpretation is probably uncertain since more recent studies have shown that after the injection of coloured polymers into a vorticose vein, it was followed by an immediate exit of the dye by the other vorticose veins, suggesting the existence of anastomosis in the drainage system [121].

Therefore, it is currently accepted that the tributary branches of the vorticose veins are very anastomosing at all levels of their branch, and there may be shunts between the watersheds of the different tributary territories.

In addition, the studies performed with fluorescein angiography indicate that experimental occlusion in monkeys in vorticose veins originate a deficit in drainage as indicated by the persistence of fluorescence in the affected quadrant. Nevertheless, the realization of the angiography a few hours later shows that there is little or no deficit in the affected area. Therefore, the restoration of the normal flow pattern in the affected area implies the existence of alternative drainage routes, which could be due to venular anastomoses.

It should also be taken into account that the macular area and the area around the optic nerve represent the areas which are most distal to the choroidal venous drainage of the vorticose veins. As a result, these are areas where the choroidal venous pressure is highest, and therefore, they are the areas which are especially sensitive to any obstruction of the venular drainage [122, 123].

Recently, it has been postulated that a paravascular transport system, which is present in the eye is analogous to the recently discovered glymphatic system in the brain. It is a functional waste clearance pathway that promotes elimination of interstitial solutes, including β-amyloid, from the brain along the paravascular channels [124]. The glymphatic system was first described by Iliff et al. (2012) [125] as a brain-wide network of paravascular channels, along which a large proportion of subarachnoid cerebrospinal fluid (CSF) recirculated through the brain parenchyma, facilitating the clearance of interstitial solutes, including β-amyloid, from the brain. This anatomical pathway consists of a para-arterial CSF influx route, a paravenous interstitial fluid clearance route and a transparenchimal pathway, which are dependent upon astroglial water transport via the astrocytic aquaporin-4 water channel [126]. Iliff et al., 2013 [127], proposed that a similar glymphatic system or, at least, a paravascular system be present in the retina. Wostyng et al. (2015) [128] suggested that the glymphatic system may also have potential clinical relevance for the understanding of the pathophysiology of glaucoma. The presence of this clearance system would support the hypothesis that glaucoma as well as Alzheimer disease and may occur when there is an imbalance between the production and clearance of neurotoxins [129]. In addition, Mathieu et al. (2017) [130] provides the first evidence that CSF flows into the optic nerve through paravascular spaces that surround small perforating pial vessels as they enter into the optic nerve. This glymphatic pathway is comprised of centripetal spaces bonded by blood vessel walls on one side and aquaporin-4+ astrocytic endfeet on the other. A dysfunction in the glymphatic system in glaucoma patients would support the hypothesis that CSF circulatory alteration may play a contributory role in glaucomatous damage.

2.3.3. Biomechanics of the laminar region

LC is believed to be the site where the main damage to the axons of the CGRs in glaucoma can occur. It is an interesting region from the biomechanical point of view, since within this site, there is a discontinuity in the corneal-scleral covering that constitutes a weak point in the mechanical load systems, and therefore, this is where the stress can be concentrated [131].

An increase in IOP can act mechanically in the tissues of the eye, producing deformations, tension and stress, which will be larger or smaller depending on the geometry and the material properties of each eye. When the levels of stress and tension exceed the physiological tolerance of the tissue cells, they can induce remodelling of the connective tissue (increase the production or eliminate collagen and elastin), in an attempt to return to a mechanical environment homeostasis [132]. This increase in the connective tissue could seriously alter the blood flow by compression of the vessels derived from the Zinn-Haller circle and therefore affect nutrition in the laminar region. It must be taken into account that this could all occur with the IOP within the normal range in those eyes, which are particularly susceptible to IOP-related stress [133, 134]. It is believed that connective tissue disorders, related to IOP, can cause the anterior lamellae of the LC to give way or be destroyed, thereby transferring the load (weight) to adjacent lamellae in a cascade of damage that would help cause, together with the loss of axons, the glaucomatous excavation [135, 136].

The LC forms a barrier between two differentially pressurized compartments: the intraocular space with higher pressure (IOP) and the retrobulbar space with a lower pressure retrobulbar cerebrospinal fluid pressure (CSFP). A pressure gradient is formed cross the LC. The pressure difference between the two compartments is denominated the translaminar pressure difference (TLPD) and is defined as IOP-CSFP. At a given IOP, subjects with a lower CSFP have a larger TLPD, which can result in the posterior deformation of the LC [137, 138]. The ability of the LC to tolerate a given TLPD without being deformed may be associated with the material properties (compliance, stiffness or structural rigidity) and geometry (thickness, shape or curvature) of the LC and the peripapillary connective tissues [135, 139]. Based on the notion that the translaminar pressure dynamics may influence LC deformation and an optic nerve axoplasmic transport, it can be speculated that eyes with a larger TLPD or translaminar pressure gradient (TLPG) may have an increased susceptibility to glaucomatous damage. Posterior deformation of the anterior LC surface is considered one of the key manifestations of glaucomatous optic neuropathy [136].

A high translaminar pressure gradient can induce the blockade of the axonal flow within the optic nerve fibres at the level of the LC [140, 141]. The TLPG may be influenced by the properties of the other structures, such as low CSFP [142–144] and a thinner LC, both of which increase the TLPG [140, 145–147]. It has been reported that a thinner central corneal thickness (CCT) is a risk factor for the conversion of ocular hypertension to primary open-angle glaucoma [148, 149] because of a thin cornea inducing a falsely low IOP measurement and a thin cornea being associated with a more susceptible optic nerve complex. However, histologic studies have found that there is no significant correlation between CCT and LC thickness [150, 151].

The deformation, the mechanical stress and the consequent increase of the collagen in the LC cause the axons to suffer deformations and mechanical stress as it passes through the pores of the LC. This can produce a mitochondrial dysfunction, which leads to a lower production of energy, triggering a blockage of the axonal transport of molecules, among which there exist neurotrophic factors (such as BDNF) which originate in the brain. These neurotrophic factors are transported towards the soma of the CGRs. The decrease of these factors, which is important for the regulation of metabolism and cell survival, can lead to the progression of the death of CGRs by apoptosis. Therefore, the alteration of the axoplasmic flow would be one of the first events that induce CGR apoptosis in glaucoma.

As we have already mentioned, the mechanical stress generated by IOP produces the reactivation of the astrocytes, causing the remodelling of the ECM. The integrins would act as mechanosensors intercommunicating the astrocytes with the ECM. In this remodelling, there is an increase in type VI and type IV collagens (the latter being a constituent of the astrocyte basement membrane) which will modify the original structure of the cribriform pores. In addition, proteoglycans and glycosaminoglycans can also be modified and the elastic fibres can degenerate. All of this leads to the biomechanical alteration of the tissue described previously.

The ECM is also responsible for providing adhesion signals, thereby controlling the functions of cells and cell survival. Reactive astrocytes increase the activity of matrix metalloproteinases (MMPs), which are enzymes involved in ECM remodelling in such a way that they can degrade cell adhesion molecules to allow cell mobility. Therefore, changes in the specific components of the ECM (increased MMP-9, laminin loss, etc.) can interrupt cell–cell and ECM-cell interactions, which could cause, in the case of CGRs, cell death by apoptosis.

Tenascins represent key constituents of the ECM with a major impact on the central nervous system development. Several studies indicated that they play a crucial role in axonal growth and guidance, synaptogenesis and boundary formation. These functions are not only important during development but also for regeneration under several pathological conditions. Tenascin C represents a key modulator in the immune system and inflammatory processes [152]. It is not only involved in barrier formation, but it is also a constituent of the glial scar after injury. Furthermore, it might be implicated in reactivation of astrocytes which play a crucial role in glaucomatous optic nerve fibrosis [153].

2.4. The retrolaminar region

This zone extends from the end of the LC to the place where the central blood vessels (CRA and central retinal vein) enter the optic nerve (**Figures 2A** and **3A**).

The retrolaminar region (RLR) is a part of the intraorbital portion of the optic nerve and, as such, is surrounded by the meningeal sheaths: dura, arachnoid and pia mater. These leave two spaces called subdural (between the dura mater and the arachnoid) and subarachnoid (between the arachnoid and the pia mater) (**Figure 9A**).

This region is distinguished by the appearance of oligodendrocytes that myelinate the axons of this zone (**Figures 3F1**, **F2** and **9C**). The bundles of axons are arranged in a polygonal shape

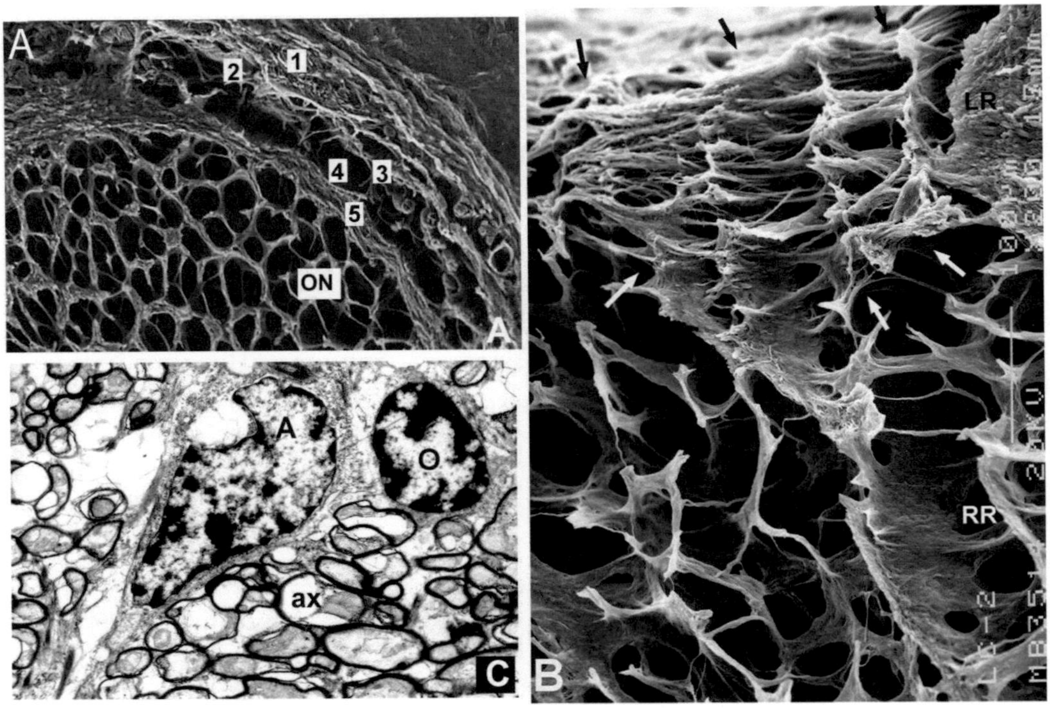

Figure 9. Retrolaminar region. (A) Meningeal sheaths surrounding the retrolaminar region of the optic nerve (ON). (1) dura mater, (2) subdural space, (3) arachnoid, (4) subarachnoid space, and (5) pia mater. (B) Connective septa. The arrows indicate the laminar region (LR). Retrolaminar region (RR). (C) Transmission electron microscopy showing the astrocytes (a), myelinated axons (ax) and oligodendrocytes (O). (A, B) scanning electron microscopy with nervous tissue digestion by trypsin. (C) Transmission electron microscopy.

and surrounded by connective tissue septa (**Figure 9B**). These septa are attached to the pia mater peripherally, to the lamina cribrosa in its anterior portion and to the connective tissue of the adventitia of the CRA in its central portion. These septa are also responsible for driving the vessels into the interior of the optic nerve [29].

Axon diameter along with myelin thickness [154], internode [155] and paranode gap [156] determines the functional properties of the nerves [157]. Axon diameter has been used to determine conduction velocity along various pathways. Thus, this indicates that there is a strong link between structure and function in the central nervous system. The characterization of ultrastructural properties of the axons has proven useful in exploring the pathology of neurological condition [155]. In the axons, the mitochondria are accumulated around the areas of highest energy demand, such as the nodes of Ranvier, in which the ATP is necessary to maintain the activity of the energetically demanding Na^+/K^+ ATPase ion pumps [158, 159]. Mitochondria change their morphology according to the energy status of the cell in processes referred to as fusion and fission [160].

2.4.1. Vascularization of the retrolaminar region

The vascularization of the optic nerve in this region varies in function of the central or peripheral location of the tissue. Thus, the axial or central zone is fundamentally nourished by the vessels coming from the CRA, while the peripheral zone receives vessels from the CRA through its pial arteries or vessels derived from the ciliary system from Zinn-Haller circle and the peripapillary choroids. In the most posterior areas, the contribution from the branches of the ophthalmic artery and its collaterals is important (**Figure 10A**) [8, 41, 43, 161].

2.4.2. Macroglia and microglia of the retrolaminar region

There are three types of glial cells in the retrolaminar region:

- Astrocytes which contribute to the fasciculation of axons and their separation from blood vessels and connective tissue. In this region, the main fasciculation of the axons is carried out by the connective septa (**Figures 3F2**, **9B** and **C**)
- Microglia which are scarce cells, but they are, in a proportion, similar to those of the rest of the optic nerve (**Figure 4C**)
- The oligodendrocytes which are responsible for the formation of the demyelin sheaths of the axons (**Figures 3F2** and **9C**)

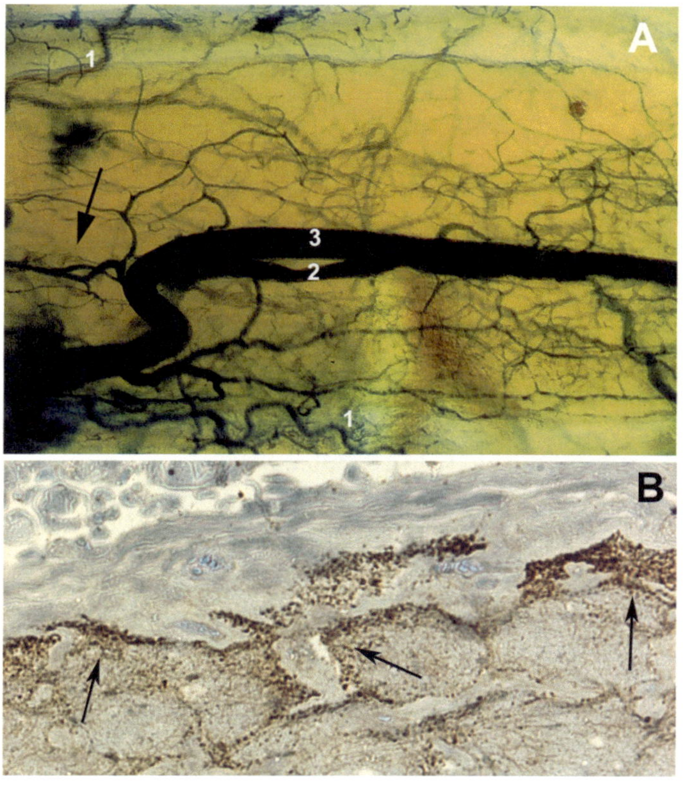

Figure 10. Retrolaminar region. (A) Vascularization: (1) pial vascularization, (2) central retinal artery, and (3) central retinal vein. (B) Peripheral glial mantle of Graefe (arrows). (A) Diaphanization technique and vascular filling with polymers. (B) Immunohistochemistry GFAP-Ünna-Tanzer.

The appearance of myelin in this area causes the thickness of the nerve to increase double in comparison to the level observed in the LC, going from 1.5 mm to 3 mm. Myelination of the nerve is necessary for the saltatory conduction of the nerve impulse. The absence of myelin can be lethal, and this has been demonstrated in animals that have a mutation in myelin proteins such as proteolipid protein (PPL) and myelin basic protein (PBM). In addition, the demyelination of axons causes neurological dysfunctions as those observed in multiple sclerosis [8].

In cell cultures, it has been shown that oligodendrocytes and astrocytes originate from a common precursor, the bipotential cells A2-B5+ [162–164]. These can generate to both a subpopulation of astrocytes called type 2 and oligodendrocytes, which is why they have been called progenitors of oligodendrocyte-type-2 astrocytes (O-2A) [164, 165].

The differentiation of progenitors O-2A into astrocyte type 2 requires environmental signals such as the interaction of a ciliary neurotrophic factor (CNTF) [166] with components of the ECM [70]. The absence of these signals generates oligodendrocytes [167, 168].

The maturation of oligodendrocyte precursors occurs in a series of stages recognized by the expression of different surface antigens, by morphological and motility characteristics and by the response to specific growth factors [169]. The precursors of the immature A2B5+ oligodendrocytes are very mobile. They have a characteristic bipolar morphology and express surface antigens which include the glycoprotein NG2 and the ganglioside GD364. As the precursor matures, it becomes less mobile and more processes appear. Although it retains its positivity for A2B5, it begins to express additional antigens, which include an antigen denominated POA [6], which is recognized by the antibody monoclonal O4 [170] (O4+ cells). At a later stage of maturation, high levels of galactocerebroside, which is the main glycolipid of myelin, are expressed [164].

The elaboration of myelin sheaths is associated with the expression of specific myelin components such as the basic myelin protein (MBP) and the proteolipid protein (PPL) [10, 171].

The proliferation of the oligodendrocyte precursor is induced by different mitogens at different stages of development. The precursor of the immature oligodendrocyte A2B5+ proliferates mainly in response to a platelet-derived growth factor (PDGF) and to a lesser extent to the growth factor of type II fibroblasts (bFGF) [172]. The precursors of the most mature oligodendrocytes O4 (+) do not respond to PDGF but retain their proliferative response to bFGF.

Experimental studies with lipophilic dyes have shown that the origin of the oligodendrocyte precursors of the optic nerve is found in the floor of the III ventricle, producing a migration from this zone to the chiasm and subsequently to the optic nerve [173]. The production of tenascin C by astrocytes regulates the migration of oligodendrocyte precursors at the level of the LC [170]. It has been suggested that glial precursors use similar molecular cues to those that guide axons during central nervous system development. These signals have been characterized as netrin-1 for oligodendrocytes and semaphorin 3a for astroglial cells [174].

The oligodendrocytes will be responsible for the formation of the myelin sheath, while the type-2 astrocytes would be in charge of the maintenance of the nodes of Ranvier, controlling the perinodal ion concentrations and providing nutrients to the axon [8]. The nodes of Ranvier are the areas of the axon where the myelin is interrupted. Its importance lies in the fact that the propagation of action potentials takes place by jumping from node to node, which leads to greater efficiency in nerve conduction. The astrocytes send perinodal processes that surround the unmyelinated axonal plasma membrane. This association suggests that it may play an important role in the physiology of the node, in such a way that specific conditions can be created to generate action potentials [175]. The astrocytes, therefore, could synthesize and renew ion channels of the nodal membrane. In addition, the sodium channels of the perinodal astrocytes could be involved in the ionic homeostasis of the perinodal space, in which the ion buffers the perinodal space dependent on the electrical activity of the node [8].

There is another cellular type in relation to nodes of Ranvier called NG2-glia. These cells express the NG2 chondroitin sulphate proteoglycan. NG2-glia share many morphological features with astrocytes but do not appear to express the conventional mature astrocyte markers (GFAP, vimentin, S-100, glutamine synthetase) and do not contain intermediate glial filaments. However, NG2-glia, in the CNS, have not only been considered to be adult oligodendrocyte progenitor cells (OPC) based on their antigenic phenotype but also to be equivalent to O-2A cells. The possible role of these cells could be to monitor and respond rapidly to changes in axonal activity, resulting in stereotypic injury response and possibly in the regeneration of remyelinating oligodendrocytes [176]. Nevertheless, other authors have found NG-2 expression in astrocytes and confirm the non-selective nature of NG-2 expression since some populations of astrocytes express the antigen [177].

In the retrolaminar region, as in the other parts of the nerve, there exists a glial tissue formed by thick bodied astrocytes, which separate the pia mater from the optic nerve axons. It is denominated the peripheral glial mantle of Graefe (**Figure 10B**). The characteristics of this glial mantle are similar to those of the other limiting glial membranes previously described in the optic nerve [29, 171, 30]. Furthermore, in these subpial astrocytes, the existence of invaginations in the plasma membranes called caveolar vesicles have been described, as well as contractile microfilaments. The function of both is to initiate the contraction of the peripheral glial mantle of Graefe in response to the stresses that may occur in the meningeal sheaths of the optic nerve [178].

2.5. Blood-central nervous system barriers

The central nervous system is a very sensitive system in the human body. Thus, the presence of specialized structures to maintain a stable ionic environment that allows correct neuronal activities and isolates the neurons from the cerebrospinal fluid and blood is necessary [179]. Based on this, capillaries of the central nervous system have tight cell junctions between endothelial cells, low numbers of pinocytic vesicles, and specific transporters (the blood-brain barrier), so that they can control fluid and molecular movement and provide a barrier effect against the leakage of materials from the capillaries [181]. In the ocular central nervous system, there are two types of blood-tissue barriers: the blood-retinal barrier (BRB) and the blood-optic nerve barrier (BONB) [181].

Molecules can be transported through barriers, but it is a highly regulated process. The molecules are transported in two ways. Firstly, the paracellular pathway is regulated by the dynamic opening and closing of the inter-endothelial junctions. Secondly, the transcellular pathway involves the formation of specialized transport vesicles (the caveolae) and the transport mediated by receptors [182, 183].

The paracellular pathway restricts the passage of solutes of more than three nm and is the preferred route for the passage of water and small water-soluble compounds [184]. The junctions between the endothelial cells are formed by tight junctions, adherent junctions and gap junctions. The tight junctions are interspersed with adherent junctions, which are formed before tight junctions favouring their formation. Gap junctions can facilitate the assembly of tight junctions and adherent junctions [182]. The main proteins of the tight junctions are the occludins and the claudins that form a barrier and regulate the permeability [185, 186]. Moreover, the ZO-1 is an adapter protein that connects to the cytoskeleton, which can participate in the contraction of the cells and therefore regulate the dynamic opening of tight junctions [187].

The transcellular pathway (or transcytosis) is the preferred route for the active transport of macromolecules. It is carried out through caveolae and transport mechanisms mediated by receptors. In hemato-nervous barriers, transcytosis is different from the endothelium, which does not form a barrier, and therefore, they have a lower number of caveolae (mainly on the side of the lumen) and express less caveolin-1, albumin receptors, and other molecules.

Other cells that regulate BRB and BONB are the pericytes, which are part of the neurovascular unit. In the retina, the relationship between endothelial cells and pericytes is 1:1 suggesting an important role of pericytes in the BRB. Pericytes are arranged around capillaries wrapped in the basal membrane and communicate with endothelial cells, macroglia (astrocytes, glia Müller), microglia and neurons. Although the basal membrane of the endothelial cells, both cells at some points separate, the pericytes make direct contact. The direct pericyte-endothelial contact is established via junctional complexes located to peg-socket contacts at sites were the basement membrane is absent [188]. The interactions between both cell types are important for the maturation, remodelling and maintenance of the vascular system through the autocrine and paracrine regulation by growth factors, as well as for basal membrane modulation [189]. During the development, the release of PDGF-B by the endothelial cells attracts the pericytes, forming tight junctions immediately after their recruitment. In addition, pericytes are able to attract glial cells [190].

The concept of the so-called neurovascular unit (NVU) is wider because the neurons and microglial cells are part of the cells involved in the blood barrier regulation. This neurovascular unit is composed of [186]:

1. The tight junctions between the endothelial cells, which restrict paracellular diffusion and effectively 'seal' the vessels
2. The continuous basal membrane that lines the endothelial cells
3. The pericytes that are embedded within this matrix, located between the endothelial cells and the astroglial endothelial feet

4. The processes of astrocytes, which communicate with the neurons and local synapses, as well as [183] cover the vessels, known as 'vascular feet'
5. Resident microglia, which can monitor its microenvironment with their processes and respond quickly to insults at or near the NVU
6. The retinal neurons

2.5.1. Blood-retinal barrier (BRB)

The internal BRB is established by the tight junctions of the endothelial cells of the retinal capillaries. These cells, which form a continuous layer, are arranged on a basement membrane, which is covered by astrocytes and the Müller cell processes, sealing the retinal capillaries. In addition, in many areas the basement membrane unfolds around pericytes. The latter do not form a continuous layer and therefore do not contribute physically to the diffusion barrier. Pericytes, astrocytes and Müller's glia can influence the activity of endothelial cells of the retina and therefore barrier properties, sending them regulatory signals (such as cytokines), which indicate changes in the microenvironment of neuronal circuits [191].

2.5.2. Blood-optic nerve barrier (BONB)

The capillaries of the optic nerve have barrier properties due to the presence of tight inter-endothelial cell junctions. In addition, in the optic nerve, the pial vessels and the Kuhnt intermediary tissue (located between the outer retinal layers and the ONH prelaminar region), which are also composed of astrocytes, also form a well-established blood-tissue barrier [181]. In the tissue of Kuhnt, the barrier consists of the tight junctions between the astrocytes of this tissue and the epithelium pigment of the retina, in addition to the desmosomes between the astrocytes and the outer limiting membrane [192]. However, the border tissue of Jacoby, which is located between the choroids and the ONH, and is composed of astrocytes, has defects in the barrier, which allows the filtration of the materials through them [192, 193]. Because the endothelial cells of the choriocapillaris have fenestrations, much of the material is freely filtered through the Jacoby border tissue to enter the prelaminar region of the optic nerve [179].

Another site where the BONB is not absolutely perfect is the prelaminar region. When a tracer was used to analyse the permeability of this region, it was observed that the prelaminar region showed a diffused distribution of the tracer in its extracellular spaces. The tracer was most concentrated in the posterior part of the prelaminar region and aggregated densely in the glial columns and around the capillaries in the ONH. The border of tissue of Jacoby was densely infiltrated. The diffusion of the tracer was less extensive in the lamina cribrosa and in the retrolaminar optic nerve region than in the prelaminar region [192, 194]. The microvessels in the prelaminar region of the ONH lacked classical barriers in the blood tissue and showed a non-specific permeability, possibly mediated by vesicular transport [195]. The absence of BONB in the prelaminar region would nullify the advantages attributed to barriers in the optic nerve blood vessels and could play a role in the development of noninflammatory optic neuropathies [180]. In the CNS there is only one other site in which there is a no blood-brain barrier, the postrema area (a small area located in the lateral wall of the fourth ventricle) [180].

Acknowledgements

The authors would like to thank Matthew Astra for correcting the English version of this work.

This work was supported by (i) the Ophthalmological Network OFTARED (RD16/0008/0005), of the Institute of Health of Carlos III of the Spanish Ministry of Economy; by the PN I+D+i 2008–2011, by the ISCIII-Subdirección General de Redes y Centros de Investigación Cooperativa; and by the European programme FEDER and (ii) SAF-2014-53779-R from the Spanish Ministry of Economy and Competitiveness. Grants to Elena Salobrar-Garcia are currently supported by a Predoctoral Fellowship (FPU13/01910) from the Spanish Ministry of Education, Culture and Sport.

Conflict of interest

The authors have no conflicts of interest to declare.

Author details

Juan J. Salazar[1,2], Ana I. Ramírez[1,2], Rosa De Hoz[1,2], Elena Salobrar-Garcia[1], Pilar Rojas[1,4], José A. Fernández-Albarral[1], Inés López-Cuenca[1], Blanca Rojas[1,3], Alberto Triviño[1,3] and José M. Ramírez[1,3]*

*Address all correspondence to: ramirezs@med.ucm.es

1 Ramon Castroviejo Institute of Ophthalmologic Research, Complutense University of Madrid (UCM), Spain

2 Department of Immunology, Ophthalmology and Otorhinolaryngology, School of Optics and Optometry, Complutense University of Madrid (UCM), Spain

3 Department of Immunology, Ophthalmology and Otorhinolaryngology, School of Medicine, Complutense University of Madrid (UCM), Spain

4 Service of Ophthalmology Hospital Gregorio Marañon, Complutense University of Madrid (UCM), Spain

References

[1] Llorca FO, editor. Anatomía Humana. Tomo II. Editorial Científico-Médica Barcelona; 1972

[2] Forrester JV, Dick AD, McMenamin PG, Roberts F, Pearlman E. The Eye: Basic Sciences in Practice. 4th ed. London: WB Saunders Ltd.; 2015. 568 p

[3] Kline LB, Bajandas FJ. Neuro-Ophthalmology Review Manual. 6th ed. Thorofare (NHJ): SLACK incorporated; 2008

[4] Trattler WB, Kaiser PK, Friedman NJ. Review of ophthalmology E-book: Expert consult-online and print. Elsevier Health Sciences. 2012

[5] Kanamori A, Nakamura M, Yamada Y, Negi A. Spectral-domain optical coherence tomography detects optic atrophy due to optic tract syndrome. Graefe's Archive for Clinical and Experimental Ophthalmology. 2013;**251**:591-595

[6] Oyster CW. The Human Eye. Structure and Function. Sunderland: Sinauer Associates Sunderland; 1999. 769 p

[7] Morrison JC. The microanatomy of the optic nerve. In: Drance SM, editor. Optic Nerve in Glaucoma. Amsterdam: Kugler Publications; 1995. pp. 57-78

[8] Ramírez J, Triviño A, Salazar J, Ramírez A. Conceptos actuales sobre la organización anatómica del nervio óptico. In: Neuritis Óptica. Madrid: Tecnomedia Editorial SL; 1997. pp. 9-28

[9] Bron AJ, Tripathi RC, Tripathi BJ. Wolff's Anatomy of the Eye and Orbit. 8th ed. London: Chapman & Hall Medical; 1997. 736 p

[10] Radius RL, Anderson DR. The course of axons through the retina and optic nerve head. Archives of Ophthalmology. 1979;**97**:1154-1158

[11] Minckler DS. The organization of nerve fibre bundles in the primate optic nerve head. Archives of Ophthalmology. 1980;**98**:1630-1636

[12] Quigley HA, Addicks EM. Quantitative studies of retinal nerve fibre layer defects. Archives of Ophthalmology. 1982;**100**:807-814

[13] Ogden TE. Nerve fibre layer of the macaque retina: Retinotopic organization. Investigative Ophthalmology & Visual Science. 1983;**24**:85-98

[14] FitzGibbon T. The human fetal retinal nerve fibre layer and optic nerve head: A DiI and DiA tracing study. Visual Neuroscience. 1997;**14**:433-447

[15] Fitzgibbon T, Taylor SF. Retinotopy of the human retinal nerve fibre layer and optic nerve head. Journal of Comparative Neurology. 1998;**375**:238-251

[16] Gupta P, Jing T, Marziliano P, Baskaran M, Cheung GC, Lamoureux EL, Cheung CY, Wong TY, Aung T, Cheng CY. Peripapillary choroidal thickness assessed using automated choroidal segmentation software in an Asian population. British Journal of Ophthalmology. 2015;**99**:920-926

[17] Huang W, Wang W, Zhou M, Chen S, Gao X, Fan Q, Ding X, Zhang X. Peripapillary choroidal thickness in healthy Chinese subjects. BMC Ophthalmology. 2013:1323-2415

[18] Ouyang Y, Heussen FM, Mokwa N, Walsh AC, Durbin MK, Keane PA, Sanchez PJ, Ruiz-Garcia H, Sadda SR. Spatial distribution of posterior pole choroidal thickness by spectral domain optical coherence tomography. Investigative Ophthalmology & Visual Science. 2011;**52**:7019-7026

[19] Tanabe H, Ito Y, Terasaki H. Choroid is thinner in inferior region of optic discs of normal eyes. Retina. 2012;**32**:134-139

[20] Ikuno Y, Kawaguchi K, Nouchi T, Yasuno Y. Choroidal thickness in healthy Japanese subjects. Investigative Ophthalmology & Visual Science. 2010;**51**:2173-2176

[21] Jonas JB, Mardin CY, Schlotzer-Schrehardt U, Naumann GO. Morphometry of the human lamina cribrosa surface. Investigative Ophthalmology & Visual Science. 1991;**32**:401-405

[22] Quigley HA, Addicks EM. Regional differences in the structure of the lamina cribrosa and their relation to glaucomatous optic nerve damage. Archives of Ophthalmology. 1981;**99**:137-143

[23] Radius RL, Gonzales M. Anatomy of the lamina cribrosa in human eyes. Archives of Ophthalmology. 1981;**99**:2159-2162

[24] Gupta P, Cheung CY, Baskaran M, Tian J, Marziliano P, Lamoureux EL, Cheung CM, Aung T, Wong TY, Cheng CY. Relationship between Peripapillary choroid and retinal nerve fiber layer thickness in a population-based sample of nonglaucomatous eyes. American Journal of Ophthalmology. 2016:1614-11.e1-2

[25] López-García C, Nácher J. Las células del tejido nervioso: Neuronas y células gliales. In: Manual de Neurociencia. Madrid: Editorial Síntesis; 1998. pp. 59-93

[26] Bunt A, Minckler D. Optic Nerve Axonal Transport: Basic Aspects. Biomedical Foundations of Ophthalmology. Philadelphia: Harper & Row; 1982. pp. 1-11

[27] Bringmann A, Pannicke T, Grosche J, Francke M, Wiedemann P, Skatchkov SN, Osborne NN, Reichenbach A. Müller cells in the healthy and diseased retina. Progress in Retinal and Eye Research. 2006;**25**:397-424

[28] Minckler DS. Optic nerve axonal transport: Clinical aspects. In: Jakobiec FA, editor. Ocular Anatomy, Embryology, and Teratology. Philadelphia: Harper & Row Publishers; 1982. pp. 650-675

[29] Triviño A, Ramírez JM, Salazar JJ, Ramírez AI, García-Sánchez J. Immunohistochemical study of human optic nerve head astroglia. Vision Research. 1996;**36**:2015-2028

[30] Triviño A, Ramírez JM, Salazar JJ, Ramírez AI. Astroglial architecture of the human optic nerve: Functional role of astrocytes. In: Castellano B, Gonzalez B, Nieto-Sampedro M, editors. Understanding Glial Cells. Boston: Kluwer Academic Publishers; 1998. pp. 63-77

[31] Ramírez JM, Triviño A, Ramírez AI, Salazar JJ, García-Sánchez J. Structural specializations of human retinal glial cells. Vision Research. 1996;**36**:2029-2036

[32] Kumpulainen T, Dahl D, Korhonen LK, Nystrom SH. Immunolabeling of carbonic anhydrase isoenzyme C and glial fibrillary acidic protein in paraffin-embedded tissue sections of human brain and retina. The Journal of Histochemistry and Cytochemistry. 1983;**31**:879-886

[33] Newman EA. A dialogue between glia and neurons in the retina: Modulation of neuronal excitability. Neuron Glia Biology. 2004;**1**:245-252

[34] Sofroniew M, Vinters H. Astrocytes: Biology and pathology. Acta Neuropathologica. 2010;**119**:7-35

[35] Kimelberg HK, Nedergaard M. Functions of astrocytes and their potential as therapeutic targets. Neurotherapeutics. 2010;**7**:338-353

[36] Nag S. Morphology and properties of astrocytes. Methods in Molecular Biology. 2011;**68**:669-100

[37] Tout S, Chan-Ling T, Hollander H, Stone J. The role of Müller cells in the formation of the blood-retinal barrier. Neuroscience. 1993;**55**:291-301

[38] Di Polo A, Aigner LJ, Dunn RJ, Bray GM, Aguayo AJ. Prolonged delivery of brain-derived neurotrophic factor by adenovirus-infected Müller cells temporarily rescues injured retinal ganglion cells. PNAS. 1998;**95**:3978-3983

[39] Dreyer EB, Zurakowski D, Schumer RA, Podos SM, Lipton SA. Elevated glutamate levels in the vitreous body of humans and monkeys with glaucoma. Archives of Ophthalmology. 1996;**114**:299-305

[40] Triviño A, Ramírez J. Anatomofisiología de la coroides. In: Gómez-Ulla F, Marín M, Ramírez JM, Triviño A, editors. La circulación coroidea. Barcelona: Edika-Med SA; 1989. pp. 7-29

[41] Ramírez J, Triviño A, Salazar J, Ramírez A. Organización microscópica de la cabeza del nervio óptico. In: Honrubia FM, García-Sánchez J, Pastor JC, editors. Diagnóstico precoz del glaucoma. Zaragoza: Talleres Gráficos Edelvives; 1997. pp. 145-179

[42] Cioffi GA, Van Buskirk EM. Vasculature of the anterior optic nerve and peripapillary choroid. In: Ritch R, Shields MB, Krupin T, editors. The Glaucomas. St. Louis: Mosby; 1996. pp. 177-188

[43] Ramírez Sebastián J, Triviño Casado A, García SJ. Vascularización de la cabeza del nervio óptico en el hombre. Archivos de la Sociedad Española de Oftalmología. 1984;**46**:413-426

[44] Hayreh S. Structure and blood supply of the optic nerve. In: Heilmann K, Richardson KT, editors. Glaucoma: Conceptions of a Disease, Pathogenesis, Diagnosis and Therapy. Stuttgart: Georg Thieme; 1978. pp. 78-96

[45] Michaelson IC. Retinal Circulation in Man and Animals. Springfield: Charles C Thomas; 1954

[46] Henkind P. Radial peripapillary capillaries of the retina. I. Anatomy: Human and comparative. The British Journal of Ophthalmology. 1967;**51**:115-123

[47] Mansoori T, Sivaswamy J, Gamalapati JS, Agraharam SG, Balakrishna N. Measurement of radial Peripapillary capillary density in the normal human retina using optical coherence tomography angiography. Journal of Glaucoma. 2017;**26**:241-246

[48] Henkind P. New observations on the radial peripapillary capillaries. Investigative Ophthalmology & Visual Science. 1967;**6**:103-108

[49] Yu PK, Cringle SJ, Yu DY. Correlation between the radial peripapillary capillaries and the retinal nerve fibre layer in the normal human retina. Experimental Eye Research. 2014;**12**:983-992

[50] Morgan WH, Hazelton ML, Azar SL, House PH, Yu DY, Cringle SJ, Balaratnasingam C. Retinal venous pulsation in glaucoma and glaucoma suspects. Ophthalmology. 2004; **111**:1489-1494

[51] Lam J, Chan G, Morgan WH, Hazelton M, Betz-Stablein B, Cringle SJ, Yu DY. Structural characteristics of the optic nerve head influencing human retinal venous pulsations. Experimental Eye Research. 2016;**145**:341-346

[52] Elkington AR, Inman CB, Steart PV, Weller RO. The structure of the lamina cribrosa of the human eye: An immunocytochemical and electron microscopical study. Eye. 1990;**4**:42-57

[53] Onda E, Cioffi GA, Bacon DR, Van Buskirk EM. Microvasculature of the human optic nerve. American Journal of Ophthalmology. 1995;**120**:92-102

[54] Ko MK, Kim DS, Ahn YK. Morphological variations of the peripapillary circle of Zinn-Haller by flat section. The British Journal of Ophthalmology. 1999;**83**:862-866

[55] Galou M, Gao J, Humbert J, Mericskay M, Li Z, Paulin D, Vicart P. The importance of intermediate filaments in the adaptation of tissues to mechanical stress: Evidence from gene knockout studies. Biology of the Cell. 1997;**89**:85-97

[56] Vazquez-Chona FR, Swan A, Ferrell WD, Jiang L, Baehr W, Chien WM, Fero M, Marc RE, Levine EM. Proliferative reactive gliosis is compatible with glial metabolic support and neuronal function. BMC Neuroscience. 2011:1298-2202-12-98

[57] Anderson DR. Fine structure and function of ocular tissues. The optic nerve. International Ophthalmology Clinics. 1973;**13**:229-242

[58] Quigley HA. Gap junctions between optic nerve head astrocytes. Investigative Ophthalmology & Visual Science. 1977;**16**:582-585

[59] Ramírez A, Salazar J, Triviño A, Solas M, Ramírez J. Las células astrogliales como constituyentes de las barreras limitantes de la cabeza del nervio óptico humano. Archivos de la Sociedad Española de Oftalmología. 1998;**73**:11-16

[60] Okinami S, Ohkuma M, Tsukahara I. Kuhnt intermediary tissue as a barrier between the optic nerve and retina. A Albrecht von Graefe's Archive for Clinical and Experimental Ophthalmology. 1976;**201**:57-67

[61] Perry VH, Bell MD, Brown HC, Matyszak MK. Inflammation in the nervous system. Current Opinion in Neurobiology. 1995;**5**:636-641

[62] Streit WJ, Walter SA, Pennell NA. Reactive microgliosis. Progress in Neurobiology. 1999;**57**:563-581

[63] de Hoz R, Gallego BI, Ramírez AI, Rojas B, Salazar JJ, Valiente-Soriano FJ, Avilés-Trigueros M, Villegas-Perez MP, Vidal-Sanz M, Triviño A. Rod-like microglia are restricted to eyes with laser-induced ocular hypertension but absent from the microglial changes in the contralateral untreated eye. PLoS One. 2013;**8**:e83733

[64] Gallego BI, Salazar JJ, de Hoz R, Rojas B, Ramírez AI, Salinas-Navarro M, Ortín-Martínez A, Valiente-Soriano FJ, Avilés-Trigueros M, Villegas-Perez MP. IOP induces upregulation of GFAP and MHC-II and microglia reactivity in mice retina contralateral to experimental glaucoma. Journal of Neuroinflammation. 2012;**9**:92

[65] Ramírez AI, Salazar JJ, de Hoz R, Rojas B, Gallego BI, Salinas-Navarro M, Alarcón-Martínez L, et al. Quantification of the effect of different levels of IOP in the astroglia of the rat retina ipsilateral and contralateral to experimental glaucoma. Investigative Ophthalmology & Visual Science. 2010;**51**:5690-5696

[66] Hernandez MR. The optic nerve head in glaucoma: Role of astrocytes in tissue remodelling. Progress in Retinal and Eye Research. 2000;**19**:297-321

[67] Neufeld AH. Microglia in the optic nerve head and the region of parapapillary chorioretinal atrophy in glaucoma. Archives of Ophthalmology. 1999;**117**:1050-1056

[68] Fujita Y, Imagawa T, Uehara M. Comparative study of the lamina cribrosa and the pial septa in the vertebrate optic nerve and their relationship to the myelinated axons. Tissue & Cell. 2000;**32**:293-301

[69] Dandona L, Quigley HA, Brown AE, Enger C. Quantitative regional structure of the normal human lamina cribrosa: A racial comparison. Archives of Ophthalmology. 1990;**108**:393-398

[70] Maeda H, Nakamura M, Yamamoto M. Morphometric features of laminar pores in lamina cribrosa observed by scanning laser ophthalmoscopy. Japanese Journal of Ophthalmology. 1999;**43**:415-421

[71] Wallace DM, O'Brien CJ. The role of lamina cribrosa cells in optic nerve head fibrosis in glaucoma. Experimental Eye Research. 2016;**142**:102-109

[72] Tovar-Vidales T, Wordinger RJ, Clark AF. Identification and localization of lamina cribrosa cells in the human optic nerve head. Experimental Eye Research. 2016;**147**:94-97

[73] Hernandez MR, Wang N, Hanley NM, Neufeld AH. Localization of collagen types I and IV mRNAs in human optic nerve head by in situ hybridization. Investigative Ophthalmology & Visual Science. 1991;**32**:2169-2177

[74] Sawaguchi S, Yue B, Fukuchi T, Iwata K, Kaiya T. Sulfated proteoglycans in the human lamina cribrosa. Investigative Ophthalmology & Visual Science. 1992;**33**:2388-2398

[75] Thale A, Tillmann B. The collagen architecture of the sclera--SEM and immunohistochemical studies. Annals of Anatomy. 1993;**175**:215-220

[76] Morgan JE. Optic nerve head structure in glaucoma: Astrocytes as mediators of axonal damage. Eye. 2000;**14**:437-444

[77] Paula JS, O'Brien C, Stamer WD. Life under pressure: The role of ocular cribriform cells in preventing glaucoma. Experimental Eye Research. 2016;**15**:1150-1159

[78] Kirwan RP, Fenerty CH, Crean J, Wordinger RJ, Clark AF, O'Brien CJ. Influence of cyclical mechanical strain on extracellular matrix gene expression in human lamina cribrosa cells in vitro. Molecular Vision. 2005:11798-11810

[79] Lambert W, Agarwal R, Howe W, Clark AF, Wordinger RJ. Neurotrophin and neurotrophin receptor expression by cells of the human lamina cribrosa. Investigative Ophthalmology & Visual Science. 2001;**42**:2315-2323

[80] Voorhees AP, Jan NJ, Austin ME, Flanagan JG, Sivak JM, Bilonick RA, Sigal IA. Lamina Cribrosa pore shape and size as predictors of neural tissue mechanical insult. Investigative Ophthalmology & Visual Science. 2017;**58**:5336-5346

[81] Jonas JB, Fernandez MC, Sturmer J. Pattern of glaucomatous neuroretinal rim loss. Ophthalmology. 1993;**100**:63-68

[82] Jonas JB, Budde WM, Panda-Jonas S. Ophthalmoscopic evaluation of the optic nerve head. Survey of Ophthalmology. 1999;**43**:293-320

[83] Quigley HA, Addicks EM, Green WR. Optic nerve damage in human glaucoma. III. Quantitative correlation of nerve fibre loss and visual field defect in glaucoma, ischemic neuropathy, papilledema, and toxic neuropathy. Archives of Ophthalmology. 1982;**100**:135-146

[84] Salazar J, Ramírez J, Andrés M, Hoz RD, Triviño A. Papel funcional de los astrocitos del nervio óptico en la fasciculación axonal. Archivos de la Sociedad Española de Oftalmología. 1998;**73**:82-86

[85] Hatten ME, Liem RK, Shelanski ML, Mason CA. Astroglia in CNS injury. Glia. 1991;**4**: 233-243

[86] Walz W, Lang MK. Immunocytochemical evidence for a distinct GFAP-negative subpopulation of astrocytes in the adult rat hippocampus. Neuroscience Letters. 1998;**257**:127-130

[87] Cunningham ET Jr, Adamis AP, Altaweel M, Aiello LP, Bressler NM, D'Amico DJ, Goldbaum M, Guyer DR, Katz B, Patel M, Schwartz SD. Macugen diabetic retinopathy

study group. A phase II randomized double-masked trial of pegaptanib, an anti-vascular endothelial growth factor aptamer, for diabetic macular edema. Ophthalmology. 2005; **112**:1747-1757

[88] Hayreh SS, Zimmerman MB. Optic disc edema in non-arteritic anterior ischemic optic neuropathy. Albrecht von Graefe's Archive for Clinical and Experimental Ophthalmology. 2007;**245**:1107-1121

[89] Hayreh SS. Non-arteritic anterior ischemic optic neuropathy: Role of systemic corticosteroid therapy. Survey of Ophthalmology. 2010;**55**:399-400 author reply 400-1

[90] Hayreh SS. Inter-individual variation in blood supply of the optic nerve head. Its importance in various ischemic disorders of the optic nerve head, and glaucoma, low-tension glaucoma and allied disorders. Documenta Ophthalmologica. 1985;**59**:217-246

[91] Hayreh SS. In vivo choroidal circulation and its watershed zones. Eye. 1990;**4**:273-289p

[92] Hayreh SS. The blood supply of the optic nerve head and the evaluation of it - myth and reality. Progress in Retinal and Eye Research. 2001;**20**:563-593

[93] Hayreh SS. Posterior ischaemic optic neuropathy: Clinical features, pathogenesis, and management. Eye. 2004;**18**:1188-1206

[94] Triviño A, Ramírez JM. Anatomofisiología de la coroides. In: Gómez-Ulla F, Marín F, Ramírez JM, Triviño A, editors. La circulación coroidea. Barcelona: EDIKA-MED. S.A; 1989. pp. 7-29

[95] Cioffi G, Granstam E, Alm A. Circulación ocular. In: Kaufman PL, Alm A, editors. Adler Fisiología del ojo (Aplicación clínica). 1st ed. Madrid: Elsevier; 2004. pp. 747-784

[96] Triviño A, Ramírez JM, García-Sánchez J. Study of the choroidal circulation in the human eye: Experimental model. In: Flower RW, editor. II Internacional Symposium on the Choroid. Maryland (USA); 1989. pp. 32-42

[97] Triviño A, Ramírez JM, García-Sánchez J. Estudio comparativo entre la vascularización coroidea del hombre y el animal de experimentación. Archivos de la Sociedad Española de Oftalmología. 1986;**5**:1305-1312

[98] Ducournau DH. A new technique for the anatomical study of the choroidal blood vessels. Ophthalmologica. 1982;**184**:190-197

[99] Hogan M, Alvarado J, Weddell J. Histology of the Human Eye. Philadelphia: Saunders; 1971

[100] Hogan MJ, Feeney L. Electron microscopy of the human choroid. III. The blood vessels. American Journal of Ophthalmology. 1961;**51**:1084-1097

[101] Feeney L, Hogan MJ. Electron microscopy of the human choroid. I. Cells and supporting structure. American Journal of Ophthalmology. 1961;**51**:1057-1072

[102] Yoneya S, Tso MO. Angioarchitecture of the human choroid. Archives of Ophthalmology. 1987;**105**:681-687

[103] Amalric P. Macular choriocapillaris pathology. In: Wessing A, editor. Choreocapillaries and Pigment Epithelium Involvements in Macular Diseases. Basel: Karger Publishers; 1981. pp. 24-31

[104] Saracco JB, Gastaud P, Legrignou B. The macular choroid. Ophthalmologica. 1984;**188**: 87-99

[105] Fryczkowski AW, Sherman MD. Scanning electron microscopy of human ocular vascular casts: The submacular choriocapillaris. Cells, Tissues, Organs. 1988;**132**:265-269

[106] Hayreh SS. Submacular choroidal vascular pattern. Experimental fluorescein fundus angiographic studies. Albrecht von Graefe's Archive for Clinical and Experimental Ophthalmology. 1974;**192**:181-196

[107] Riva CE, Cranstoun SD, Grunwald JE, Petrig BL. Choroidal blood flow in the foveal region of the human ocular fundus. Investigative Ophthalmology & Visual Science. 1994;**35**:4273-4281

[108] Alm A, Bill A. Ocular and optic nerve blood flow at normal and increased intraocular pressures in monkeys (Macaca irus): A study with radioactively labelled microspheres including flow determinations in brain and some other tissues. Experimental Eye Research. 1973;**15**:15-29

[109] Ramírez J, Triviño A, García Franco C, García SJ. Estudio de la vascularización coroidea por el método de diafanización. Archivos de la Sociedad Española de Oftalmología. 1984;**46**:155-160

[110] Risco JM, Grimson BS, Johnson PT. Angioarchitecture of the ciliary artery circulation of the posterior pole. Archives of Ophthalmology. 1981;**99**:864-868

[111] Hayreh SS. In vivo choroidal circulation and its watershed zones. Eye. 1990;**4**:273-289

[112] Hayreh SS. Segmental nature of the choroidal vasculature. The British Journal of Ophthalmology. 1975;**59**:631-648

[113] Hayreh SS. The long posterior ciliary arteries. An experimental study. Albrecht von Graefe's Archive for Clinical and Experimental Ophthalmology. 1974;**192**:197-213

[114] Hayreh SS. Anatomy and physiology of the optic nerve head. Transactions of the American Academy of Ophthalmology and Otolaryngology. 1974;**78**:240-254

[115] Hayreh SS. Controversies on submacular choroidal circulation. Ophthalmologica. Journal International d'Ophtalmologie. 1981;**183**:11-19

[116] Hayreh SS. The choriocapillaris. Albrecht von Graefe's Archive for Clinical and Experimental Ophthalmology. 1974;**192**:165-179

[117] Buggage R, Torcynski E, Grossniklaus HE. The uveal tract. In: Duane TD, Jaeger EA, editors. Biomedical Foundations of Ophathalmology. CD-Rom. Edición; 2004

[118] Tazzi A. Morphological remarks concerning the venous circulation of the uveal tract (author's transl). Journal Français d'Ophtalmologie. 1978;**1**:185-189

[119] Study of the choroidal circulation in the human eye: experimental model. In: Flower RW, editor. II Internacional Symposium on the Choroid. Maryland (USA); 1989

[120] Hayreh SS, Baines JA. Occlusion of the vortex veins. An experimental study. The British Journal of Ophthalmology. 1973;**57**:217-238

[121] Carella E, Carella G. Microangioarchitecture of the coroidal circulation using latex casts. In: Yanuzzi LA, Flower RW, Slakter JS, editors. Indocyanine Green Angiography. St. Louis: Mosby; 1997. pp. 24-28

[122] Friedman E. The role of the atherosclerotic process in the pathogenesis of age-related macular degeneration. American Journal of Ophthalmology. 2000;**130**:658-663

[123] Friedman E, Ivry M, Ebert E, Glynn R, Gragoudas E, Seddon J. Increased scleral rigidity and age-related macular degeneration. Ophthalmology. 1989;**96**:104-108

[124] Wostyn P, Killer HE, De Deyn PP. Glymphatic stasis at the site of the lamina cribrosa as a potential mechanism underlying open-angle glaucoma. Clinical & Experimental Ophthalmology. 2017;**45**:539-547

[125] Iliff JJ, Wang M, Liao Y, Plogg BA, Peng W, Gundersen GA, Benveniste H, Vates GE, Deane R, Goldman SA, Nagelhus EA, Nedergaard M. A paravascular pathway facilitates CSF flow through the brain parenchyma and the clearance of interstitial solutes, including amyloid beta. Science Translational Medicine. 2012;**4**:147ra111

[126] Denniston AK, Keane PA. Paravascular pathways in the eye: Is there an 'Ocular Glymphatic system? Investigative Ophthalmology & Visual Science. 2015;**56**:3955-3956

[127] Iliff JJ, Lee H, Yu M, Feng T, Logan J, Nedergaard M, Benveniste H. Brain-wide pathway for waste clearance captured by contrast-enhanced MRI. The Journal of Clinical Investigation. 2013;**123**:1299-1309

[128] Wostyn P, Van Dam D, Audenaert K, Killer HE, De Deyn PP, De Groot V. A new glaucoma hypothesis: A role of glymphatic system dysfunction. Fluids and Barriers of the CNS. 2015;**12**:16-015-0012-z

[129] Wostyn P, De Groot V, Van Dam D, Audenaert K, Killer HE, De Deyn PP. Glaucoma considered as an imbalance between production and clearance of neurotoxins. Investigative Ophthalmology & Visual Science. 2014;**55**:5351-5352

[130] Mathieu E, Gupta N, Ahari A, Zhou X, Hanna J, Yucel YH. Evidence for cerebrospinal fluid entry into the optic nerve via a Glymphatic pathway. Investigative Ophthalmology & Visual Science. 2017;**58**:4784-4791

[131] Crawford Downs J, Roberts MD, Sigal IA. Glaucomatous cupping of the lamina cribrosa: A review of the evidence for active progressive remodelling as a mechanism. Experimental Eye Research. 2011;**93**:133-140

[132] Grytz R, Meschke G, Jonas JB. The collagen fibril architecture in the lamina cribrosa and peripapillary sclera predicted by a computational remodelling approach. Biomechanics and Modeling in Mechanobiology. 2011;**10**:371-382

[133] Downs JC, Roberts MD, Burgoyne CF. Mechanical environment of the optic nerve head in glaucoma. Optometry and Vision Science. 2008;**85**:425-435

[134] Sigal IA, Bilonick RA, Kagemann L, Wollstein G, Ishikawa H, Schuman JS, Grimm JL. The optic nerve head as a robust biomechanical system. Investigative Ophthalmology & Visual Science. 2012;**53**(6):2658-2667

[135] Burgoyne CF, Downs JC, Bellezza AJ, Suh JK, Hart RT. The optic nerve head as a biomechanical structure: A new paradigm for understanding the role of IOP-related stress and strain in the pathophysiology of glaucomatous optic nerve head damage. Progress in Retinal and Eye Research. 2005;**24**(1):39-73

[136] Burgoyne CF. A biomechanical paradigm for axonal insult within the optic nerve head in aging and glaucoma. Experimental Eye Research. 2011;**93**:120-132

[137] Morgan WH, Yu DY, Alder VA, Cringle SJ, Cooper RL, House PH, Constable IJ. The correlation between cerebrospinal fluid pressure and retrolaminar tissue pressure. Investigative Ophthalmology & Visual Science. 1998;**39**:1419-1428

[138] Lee DS, Lee EJ, Kim TW, Park YH, Kim J, Lee JW, Kim S. Influence of translaminar pressure dynamics on the position of the anterior lamina cribrosa surface. Investigative Ophthalmology & Visual Science. 2015;**56**:2833-2841

[139] Pena JDO, Agapova O, Gabelt BT, Levin LA, Lucarelli MJ, Kaufman PL, Hernandez MR. Increased elastin expression in astrocytes of the lamina cribrosa in response to elevated intraocular pressure. Investigative Ophthalmology & Visual Science. 2001;**42**:2303-2314

[140] Sigal IA, Flanagan JG, Tertinegg I, Ethier CR. Modeling individual-specific human optic nerve head biomechanics. Part I: IOP-induced deformations and influence of geometry. Biomechanics and Modeling in Mechanobiology. 2009;**8**:85-98

[141] Sigal IA, Flanagan JG, Tertinegg I, Ethier CR. Predicted extension, compression and shearing of optic nerve head tissues. Experimental Eye Research. 2007;**85**:312-322

[142] Morgan WH, Chauhan BC, Yu DY, Cringle SJ, Alder VA, House PH. Optic disc movement with variations in intraocular and cerebrospinal fluid pressure. Investigative Ophthalmology & Visual Science. 2002;**43**:3236-3242

[143] Jonas JB, Berenshtein E, Holbach L. Anatomic relationship between lamina cribrosa, intraocular space, and cerebrospinal fluid space. Investigative Ophthalmology & Visual Science. 2003;**44**:5189-5195

[144] Berdahl JP, Allingham RR, Johnson DH. Cerebrospinal fluid pressure is decreased in primary open-angle glaucoma. Ophthalmology. 2008;**11**:763-768

[145] Albon J, Purslow PP, Karwatowski WS, Easty DL. Age related compliance of the lamina cribrosa in human eyes. The British Journal of Ophthalmology. 2000;**84**(3):318-323

[146] Sigal IA, Ethier CR. Biomechanics of the optic nerve head. Experimental Eye Research. 2009;**88**:799-807

[147] Ren R, Wang N, Li B, Li L, Gao F, Xu X, Jonas JB. Lamina cribrosa and peripapillary sclera histomorphometry in normal and advanced glaucomatous Chinese eyes with various axial length. Investigative Ophthalmology & Visual Science. 2009;**50**:2175-2184

[148] Gordon MO, Beiser JA, Brandt JD, Heuer DK, Higginbotham EJ, Johnson CA, Keltner JL, Miller JP, Parrish RK 2nd, Wilson MR, Kass MA. The ocular hypertension treatment study: Baseline factors that predict the onset of primary open-angle glaucoma. Archives of Ophthalmology. 2002;**120**:714-720

[149] Herndon LW, Weizer JS, Stinnett SS. Central corneal thickness as a risk factor for advanced glaucoma damage. Archives of Ophthalmology. 2004;**122**:17-21

[150] Ren R, Li B, Gao F, Li L, Xu X, Wang N, Jonas JB. Central corneal thickness, lamina cribrosa and peripapillary scleral histomorphometry in non-glaucomatous Chinese eyes. Albrecht von Graefe's Archive for Clinical and Experimental Ophthalmology. 2010;**248**:1579-1585

[151] Jonas JB, Hayreh SS, Tao Y. Central corneal thickness and thickness of the lamina cribrosa and peripapillary sclera in monkeys. Archives of Ophthalmology. 2009;**127**:1395-1396

[152] Reinhard J, Roll L, Faissner A. Tenascins in retinal and optic nerve neurodegeneration. Frontiers in Integrative Neuroscience. 2017;**1130**

[153] Schneider M, Fuchshofer R. The role of astrocytes in optic nerve head fibrosis in glaucoma. Experimental Eye Research. 2016;**14**:249-255

[154] Smith RS, Koles ZJ. Myelinated nerve fibers: Computed effect of myelin thickness on conduction velocity. The American Journal of Physiology. 1970;**219**:1256-1258

[155] Waxman SG. Determinants of conduction velocity in myelinated nerve fibers. Muscle & Nerve. 1980;**3**:141-150

[156] Arancibia-Carcamo IL, Ford MC, Cossell L, Ishida K, Tohyama K, Attwell D. Node of Ranvier length as a potential regulator of myelinated axon conduction speed. eLife. 2017; 610.7554/eLife.23329

[157] Giacci MK, Bartlett CA, Huynh M, Kilburn MR, Dunlop SA, Fitzgerald M. Three dimensional electron microscopy reveals changing axonal and myelin morphology along normal and partially injured optic nerves. Scientific Reports. 2018;**8**:3979-018-22361-2

[158] Bros H, Millward JM, Paul F, Niesner R, Infante-Duarte C. Oxidative damage to mitochondria at the nodes of Ranvier precedes axon degeneration in ex vivo transected axons. Experimental Neurology. 2014;**26**:1127-1135

[159] Aiello GL, Bach-y-Rita P. The cost of an action potential. Journal of Neuroscience Methods. 2000;**103**:145-149

[160] Chen H, Chan DC. Mitochondrial dynamics—Fusion, fission, movement, and mitophagy—In neurodegenerative diseases. Human Molecular Genetics. 2009;**18**:R169-R176

[161] Ramírez J, Triviño A. Anatomofisiología del nervio óptico. In: Gómez-Ulla F, Marín F, Ramírez JM, Triviño A, editors. La circulación coroidea. Barcelona: EDIKA-MED. S.A; 1989. pp. 31-40

[162] Hayreh SS. The sheath of the optic nerve. Ophthalmologica. 1984;**189**:54-63

[163] Pinazo-Duran M, Renau-Piqueras J, Lindo L, Guerri C. Estudio estructural de la gliogénesis, mielinización y desarrollo axonal en el nervio óptico de la rata. Archivos de la Sociedad Española de Oftalmología. 1994;**67**:13-19

[164] Miller RH, Hayes JE, Dyer KL, Sussman CR. Mechanisms of oligodendrocyte commitment in the vertebrate CNS. International Journal of Developmental Neuroscience. 1999;**17**:753-763

[165] Raff MC. Glial cell diversification in the rat optic nerve. Science. 1989;**243**:1450-1455

[166] Hughes SM, Lillien LE, Raff MC, Rohrer H, Sendtner M. Ciliary neurotrophic factor induces type-2 astrocyte differentiation in culture. Nature. 1988;**335**:70-73

[167] Quigley HA, Anderson DR. Distribution of axonal transport blockade by acute intraocular pressure elevation in the primate optic nerve head. Investigative Ophthalmology & Visual Science. 1977;**16**:640-644

[168] Miller RH, Ffrench-Constant C, Raff MC. The mCRAoglial cells of the rat optic nerve. Annual Review of Neuroscience. 1989;**12**:517-534

[169] Pfeiffer SE, Warrington AE, Bansal R. The oligodendrocyte and its many cellular processes. Trends in Cell Biology. 1993;**3**:191-197

[170] Morcos Y, Chan-Ling T. Concentration of astrocytic filaments at the retinal optic nerve junction is coincident with the absence of intra-retinal myelination: Comparative and developmental evidence. Journal of Neurocytology. 2000;**29**:665-678

[171] Ramírez A, Salazar J, Triviño A, Solas M, Ramírez J. Las células astrogliales Como constituyentes de las barreras limitantes de la cabeza del nervio óptico humano. Archivos de la Sociedad Española de Oftalmología. 1998;**73**:11-16

[172] Hernandez MR, Igoe F, Neufeld AH. Extracellular matrix of the human optic nerve head. American Journal of Ophthalmology. 1986;**102**:139-148

[173] Morgan WH, Yu DY, Cooper RL, Alder VA, Cringle SJ, Constable IJ. The influence of cerebrospinal fluid pressure on the lamina cribrosa tissue pressure gradient. Investigative Ophthalmology & Visual Science. 1995;**36**(6):1163-1172

[174] Tsai HH, Miller RH. Glial cell migration directed by axon guidance cues. Trends in Neurosciences. 2002;**25**:173-175

[175] Hildebrand C, Waxman SG. Postnatal differentiation of rat optic nerve fibers: Electron microscopic observations on the development of nodes of Ranvier and axoglial relations. The Journal of Comparative Neurology. 1984;**224**:25-37

[176] Butt AM, Pugh M, Hubbard P, James G. Functions of optic nerve glia: Axoglial signalling in physiology and pathology. Eye. 2004;**18**:1110-1121

[177] Alghamdi B, Fern R. Phenotype overlap in glial cell populations: Astroglia, oligodendroglia and NG-2(+) cells. Frontiers in Neuroanatomy. 2015 May;**12**:949

[178] Massa PT. Plasmalemmal vesicles (caveolae) of fibrous astrocytes of the cat optic nerve. The American Journal of Anatomy. 1982;**165**(1):69-81

[179] Grieshaber MC, Flammer J. Does the blood-brain barrier play a role in Glaucoma? Survey of Ophthalmology. 2007;**52**(6, Supplement 1):S115-S121

[180] Hayreh SS. Blood-optic nerve barrier. In: Hayreh SS, editor. Ischemic Optic Neuropathies. Berlin: Springer-Verlag; 2011. pp. 79-84

[181] Ramírez JM, Rojas B, Gallego BI, García-Martín ES, Triviño A, Ramírez AI, Salazar JJ, de Hoz R. Glia and Blood-Retinal Barrier: Effects of Ocular Hypertension. Hong Kong: iConcept Press; 2014. pp. 123-162

[182] Klaassen I, Van Noorden CJF, Schlingemann RO. Molecular basis of the inner blood-retinal barrier and its breakdown in diabetic macular edema and other pathological conditions. Progress in Retinal and Eye Research. 2013;**34**:19-48

[183] Diaz-Coranguez M, Ramos C, Antonetti DA. The inner blood-retinal barrier: Cellular basis and development. Vision Research. 2017;**139**:123-137

[184] Pappenheimer JR, Renkin EM, Borrero LM. Filtration, diffusion and molecular sieving through peripheral capillary membranes; a contribution to the pore theory of capillary permeability. The American Journal of Physiology. 1951;**167**:13-46

[185] Campbell M, Cassidy PS, O'Callaghan J, Crosbie DE, Humphries P. Manipulating ocular endothelial tight junctions: Applications in treatment of retinal disease pathology and ocular hypertension. Progress in Retinal and Eye Research. 2018 Jan:62120-62133

[186] Chiba H, Osanai M, Murata M, Kojima T, Sawada N. Transmembrane proteins of tight junctions. Biochimica et Biophysica Acta. 1778;**2008**:588-600

[187] Bauer H, Zweimueller-Mayer J, Steinbacher P, Lametschwandtner A, Bauer HC. The dual role of zonula occludens (ZO) proteins. Journal of Biomedicine & Biotechnology. 2010;**20**:1040-2593

[188] van Dijk CG, Nieuweboer FE, Pei JY, Xu YJ, Burgisser P, van Mulligen E, el Azzouzi H, Duncker DJ, Verhaar MC, Cheng C. The complex mural cell: Pericyte function in health and disease. International Journal of Cardiology. 2015;**190**:75-89

[189] Trost A, Lange S, Schroedl F, Bruckner D, Motloch KA, Bogner B, Kaser-Eichberger A, Strohmaier C, Runge C, Aigner L, Rivera FJ, Reitsamer HA. Brain and retinal pericytes: Origin, function and role. Frontiers in Cellular Neuroscience. 2016;**1020**

[190] Gerhardt H, Betsholtz C. Endothelial-pericyte interactions in angiogenesis. Cell and Tissue Research. 2003;**314**:15-23

[191] Abbott NJ, Patabendige AAK, Dolman DEM, Yusof SR, Begley DJ. Structure and function of the blood–brain barrier. Neurobiology of Disease. 2010;**1**(37):13-25

[192] Tso MO, Shih CY, McLean IW. Is there a blood-brain barrier at the optic nerve head? Archives of Ophthalmology. 1975;**93**:815-825

[193] Cohen AI. Is there a potential defect in the blood-retinal barrier at the choroidal level of the optic nerve canal? Investigative Ophthalmology. 1973;**12**:513-519

[194] Tsukahara I, Yamashita H. An electron microscopic study on the blood-optic nerve and fluid-optic nerve barrier. Albrecht von Graefe's Archive for Clinical and Experimental Ophthalmology. 1975;**196**:239-246

[195] Hofman P, Hoyng P, van der Werf F, Vrensen GF, Schlingemann RO. Lack of blood-brain barrier properties in microvessels of the prelaminar optic nerve head. Investigative Ophthalmology & Visual Science. 2001;**42**:895-901

Chapter 3

Optic Nerve: Developmental Anomalies and Common Tumors

Hind Alkatan, Daniah Alshowaeir and
Tariq Alzahem

Additional information is available at the end of the chapter

http://dx.doi.org/10.5772/intechopen.80326

Abstract

The optic nerve, also known as the second cranial nerve, is composed of axons that transmit visual information from the neurosensory retina to the visual cortex. There are multiple pathologies that can affect the human optic nerve. Congenital anomalies of the optic nerve include myelinated nerve fibers, morning glory syndrome, optic nerve choristoma, optic nerve coloboma, optic nerve hypoplasia and aplasia, and others. Tumors that can affect the optic nerve (ON) may occur primarily from within the nerve itself, from the surrounding optic nerve sheath (ONS), or secondarily spreading to the nerve from a distant site. They include optic pathway glioma, medulloepithelioma, oligodendroglioma, optic nerve sheath meningioma, and others. Here in this chapter, we will review the optic nerve anatomy, embryology, and physiology in addition to assessment of optic nerve function. Moreover, the clinical features, imaging findings, pathology, and treatment options of the most common and some rare congenital anomalies and primary tumors of the ON and sheath will be reviewed.

Keywords: myelinated nerve fibers, morning glory syndrome, optic nerve choristoma, optic nerve coloboma, optic nerve hypoplasia, aplasia, optic nerve tumor, glioma, meningioma, ganglioglioma, medulloepithelioma, hemangioblastoma, oligodendroglioma

1. Introduction

Visual perception occurs when light stimulus in the surrounding environment converts to nerve impulses at the level of photoreceptors, which then reach the brain to be processed. The light energy is converted to neuronal signals that are transmitted through several layers in the retina to reach the ganglion cells. The axons of the ganglion cells form the optic nerve. Signals are carried out from the optic nerve through the optic chiasm and optic tract, which is connected to the lateral geniculate body. From there, signals reach the visual cortex in the occipital lobe through the optic radiation.

The chapter is divided into three main sections. Section 1 describes the basic embryology, anatomy, and physiology of the optic nerve. Section 2 briefly discusses optic nerve developmental anomalies, and the last section briefly reviews the most common optic nerve tumors and discusses their management modalities.

2. Optic nerve embryology, anatomy, physiology, and function

2.1. Optic nerve embryology

The optic nerve has a neural ectoderm origin. It develops within the optic stalk, which appears by 22–28 days of gestation. The optic stalk connects the optic vesicle to the cavity of the forebrain [1]. It has two layers, the inner layer is the axons of the ganglion cell layer and the outer layer is a neuroglial supporting cells. At 8 weeks of gestation, neuroepithelial cells including astrocytes and oligodendrocytes proliferate and participate in the formation of the connective tissue and myelination of the optic nerve. Myelination starts centrally and reaches the lamina cribrosa at or shortly after birth [2].

2.2. Optic nerve anatomy and physiology

The nerve fiber layer in the retina is the ganglion cell axons, which are generally unmyelinated and receive blood supply from the central retinal artery. Ganglion cell axons turn 90° to enter the optic disc, where they form the optic nerve. The optic disc is supplied by a ring of branches from the short ciliary arteries called the circle of Zinn. Peripapillary arteries also contribute to the optic disc blood supply. The optic nerve consists of 1.2 million fibers with different sizes of diameter, ranging from 0.7 to 10 μm. Smaller fibers serve the central vision, while larger ones come from the peripheral retina [3]. The macular fibers are deep in the center of the optic nerve, while the fibers of the peripheral retina are more superficial.

The length of the optic nerve is around 6 cm and can be divided anatomically into four segments: intraocular (0.7–1 mm), intraorbital (30 mm), intracanalicular (6–10 mm), and intracranial (10–16 mm). The lamina cribrosa divides the intraocular part into prelaminar and laminar sections [4]. It is important to note that this part of the nerve is not myelinated. Oligodendrocytes are responsible for the myelination of nerves, and it is believed that the lamina cribrosa acts as a barrier preventing them from myelinating the intraocular section of the optic nerve [5].

Beyond the lamina cribrosa, the optic nerve is myelinated and surrounded by a dural sheath and cerebrospinal fluid. The extraocular muscles surround the optic nerve in the orbit. The optic nerve sheet is adherent to the superior and medial rectus muscle, hence the pain with eye movement when the optic nerve is inflamed in cases such as optic neuritis. The ophthalmic artery is the first branch from the internal carotid artery, and it forms the main blood supply for intraorbital and intracanalicular division of the optic nerve. The ophthalmic artery passes through the dural sheath of the optic nerve in the intracanalicular section. The intracranial optic nerve division is supplied by branches from the ophthalmic, interior cerebral, anterior communicating, and internal carotid arteries. Ninety percent of the optic nerve fibers from both sides join in the optic chiasm, while the remaining 10% of fibers project to areas controlling pupillary responses [5].

2.3. Assessment of optic nerve function

The optic nerve function is assessed by evaluating several elements including the visual acuity, color vision and contrast testing, relative afferent pupillary defect in cases of asymmetric optic neuropathy, and visual field testing. These parameters should be evaluated in every patient with suspected optic neuropathy. In addition, electrophysiological testing is another adjunctive test used to assess optic neuropathies.

2.3.1. Visual acuity (VA)

Visual acuity is a vital function of the optic nerve and an important measure of the visual function. The smallest visual angle at which two distinct objects can be distinguished is referred to as the minimum separable threshold. The best-corrected visual acuity (BCVA) should be obtained with refraction to exclude any refractive errors. The physician can expect a refractive error when there is an improvement of visual acuity with pinhole viewing.

Snellen acuity is measured with test letters (optotypes), and they are designed in a way so that the letter as a whole subtends an angle of 5 min of arc at a specified distance. A 20/40 Snellen acuity (6/12 in m) means that the patient can see the 20/40 line 20 feet away from the chart what a normal person can see clearly 40 feet away.

2.3.2. Color vision

Optic nerve diseases, especially optic neuritis, may disproportionately affect color vision compared with BCVA. In macular disease, however, both visual acuity and color vision tend to be affected congruently. In addition, color vision deficit (dyschromatopsia) can persist even after recovery of visual acuity in optic neuropathy.

Color vision testing is done monocularly. Pseudoisochromatic color plate is widely available and frequently used to evaluate color vision. Bilateral, symmetric, color vision deficit in males may indicate congenital dyschromatopsia. The most detailed color vision test is the Farnsworth-Munsell 100-hue test. It uses 85 colored discs, and thus, it needs a considerable amount of time that limits its use in routine clinical practice.

2.3.3. Contrast sensitivity

Contrast sensitivity is simply defined as the ability to recognize the degree of contrast between the optotype and its background. The higher the contrast, the easier the optotype is to be seen. Increasing the illumination makes it easier to read because this creates a higher contrast against the black letters. Snellen acuity optotypes are projecting at approximately

100% contrast that can be resolved more easily by the visual system. However, 100% contrast is rarely encountered in everyday life, and therefore, 20/20 vision does not always mean good vision as low-contrast sensitivity may significantly compromise the visual quality.

Contrast sensitivity testing can detect and quantify vision loss in the presence of normal visual acuity. The Pelli-Robson contrast sensitivity letter consists of rows of letters of equal size but with decreasing contrast for groups of three letters. Sinusoidal gratings require the test subject to view a sequence of increasingly lower contrast gratings. Many conditions reduce contrast sensitivity. They include optic neuropathy, posterior subcapsular cataracts, and amblyopia. Contrast sensitivity testing is not commonly used in clinical practice.

2.3.4. Pupillary examination

Pupillary examination and particularly testing for relative afferent pupillary defect (RAPD) is highly sensitive for optic nerve diseases. Under normal conditions, light source directed at one pupil causes symmetric ipsilateral and contralateral pupillary constriction (direct and consensual response). When the optic nerve of one eye is damaged or inflamed more than the other eye, a relative afferent pupillary defect is seen in the more affected eye. In other words, shining the light over the normal, or less affected, eye will result in bilateral pupillary constriction. However, when the light is swung to the more affected eye, we will see a bilateral pupillary dilation as the signal conduction along the optic nerve is relatively compromised compared to the other eye.

An absence of RAPD usually indicates a bilaterally normal optic nerves or a bilateral symmetric optic neuropathy. RAPD can be seen in patients with significant retinal dysfunction including central retinal artery occlusion, ischemic central retinal vein occlusion, or retinal detachment.

2.3.5. Visual field

Visual field is another important function of the optic nerve in which a visual field defect testing can describe, quantify, monitor, and localize the different patterns of visual loss. There are different techniques available to evaluate visual field. The choice of technique depends on the degree of detail required and the cooperation of the patient.

Confrontation visual field testing is a simple test that can be done at the bedside or in the clinic providing a gross evaluation of the visual fields. The examiner sits 1 m from the patient. The patient is asked to cover one eye and fixate on the examiner's nose by the other eye. Then, the examiner requests the patient to identify the numbers (1, 2, or 5) presented by the examiner's fingers at the midpoint of each of the four quadrants for each eye.

A more detailed evaluation of the visual field is assessed by perimetry. There are two main types: static and kinetic perimetry. In static testing, stimuli are static and turn on and off at different points within area the visual field to be tested. In kinetic testing, a stimulus is moved from a nonseeing peripheral area to a seeing area of the visual field. In kinetic testing, an isopter is drawn by connecting all points of equal sensitivity for a specific stimulus.

http://dx.doi.org/10.5772/intechopen.80326

2.3.6. Visual evoked potentials (VEP) in the assessment of optic nerve function

Visual evoked potential (VEP) is an electrical response recorded mainly from the visual cortex in response to light stimulus. It was first introduced in 1930s, and its role has evolved over the years [6]. In 1961, Ciganek was the first to describe an electroencephalography (EEG) response to a flashlight stimulus in humans, followed by one of the earliest clinical studies of VEP reported by Halliday and colleagues on patients with optic neuritis [7, 8].

VEP provides an objective and reproducible measure of visual function and continues to have an imperative complementary role to other tests that provide information on the structure of the visual system such as MRI and optical coherence tomography (OCT).

The recording of VEP is performed using occipital mounted electrodes with, typically, monocular stimulation. Several forms of visual stimulus can be used to generate a VEP. The most common stimuli used are flash visual evoked potential (fVEP), pattern-onset VEP, and reversing black and white checkerboard pattern (PVEP). Because of fVEP's high intersubject variability and low sensitivity, PVEP is preferred in most clinical sitting. fVEP is frequently used in infants, uncooperative patients or if significant media opacity is present. The pattern-onset VEP is preferred in patients with fixation instability such as nystagmus since the PVEP is severely reduced in those patients due to the effect of retinal image motion on the stimulus efficiency [9, 10].

The testing technique for both stimulus conditions has been standardized by the International Society of Clinical Electrophysiology of Vision (ISCEV) to reach a better consistency of results between different electrophysiology laboratories [11]. The PVEP waveform is triphasic with a prominent positive peak (P100) at around 100 ms, an earlier negative peak at around 75 ms, and a late negative peak at around 135 ms after stimulation (**Figure 1**). The amplitude of the P100 reflects the number of functional afferent axons reaching the cortex. The implicit time (latency) is believed to reflect the degree of demyelination. An abnormal VEP response

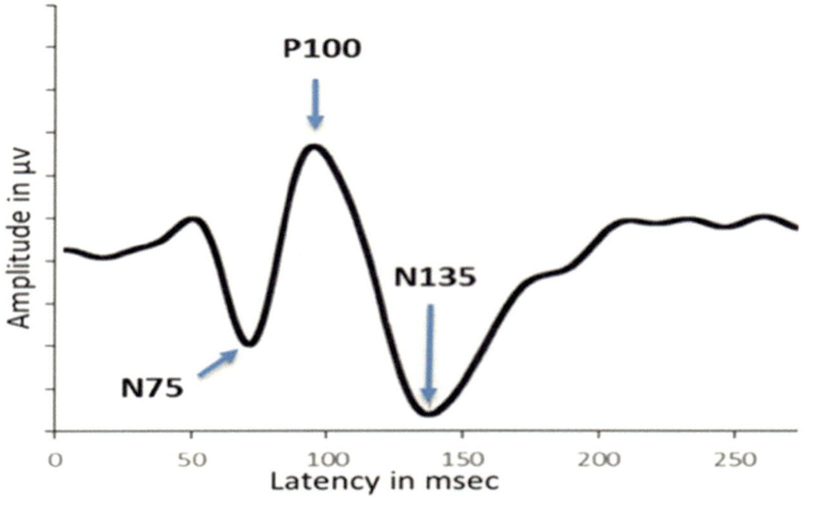

Figure 1. Normal waveform of a standard PVEP. Arrows showing first negative peak (N75), positive peak (P100), and a late negative peak (N135).

indicates a functional disturbance in the afferent visual pathway, and occasionally, conventional VEP may provide some information on the location of the lesion [12]. For example, based on the neuroanatomy of the visual system, a unilateral VEP abnormality implies an abnormality in the anterior optic pathway. Localization is less likely when the delay is bilateral.

3. Developmental anomalies of the optic nerve

3.1. Myelinated nerve fibers

The prevalence of myelinated nerve fibers (MNF) is around 1% in autopsy studies [13]. MNF are typically congenital, and therefore likely represent anomalies of myelination control in utero. They appear as gray or white striated patches with feathered borders, which are most commonly unilateral, with only 7.7% of cases estimated to occur bilaterally (**Figure 2**) [13, 14]. The mechanism by which MNF occur might be linked to unknown level of communication between adjacent oligodendrocytes (which are responsible for myelinating the axons of subsets of neurons in the central nervous system) in the selection of axons for myelination [15]. Recently, a case of bilateral extensive peripapillary MNF has been reported in a patient with Crouzon syndrome, an inherited form of craniosynostosis caused by over-activation of fibroblast growth factor receptor 2 [16].

3.2. Morning glory syndrome (MGS)

MGS is a rare congenital optic disc anomaly, first reported by Pendler [17] then more accurately described 10 years later [18]. The pathogenesis of MGS is uncertain, but probably is an embryological form of optic disc dysplasia and is thought not to be a true coloboma, but rather a posterior ectasia, which is the consequence of developmental disturbance of sclera [19, 20]. MGS is characterized by a funnel-shaped enlarged optic disc with a central mass of glial tissue and emerging radial retinal vessels that emerge from the central core toward the peripheral retina (**Figure 3**) [21]. MGS is a nonprogressive and untreatable condition, which

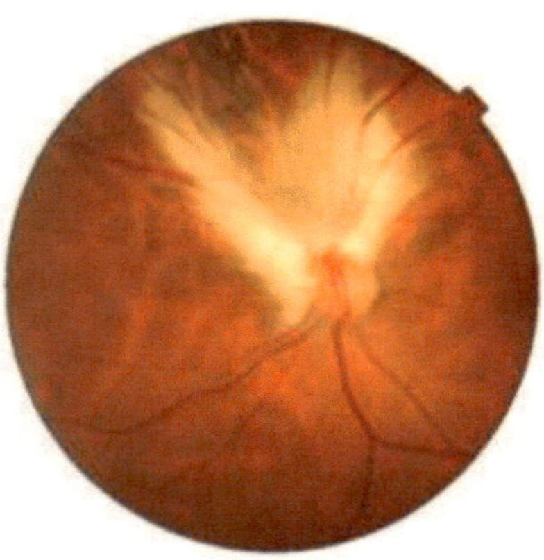

Figure 2. Myelinated nerve fibers (MNF).

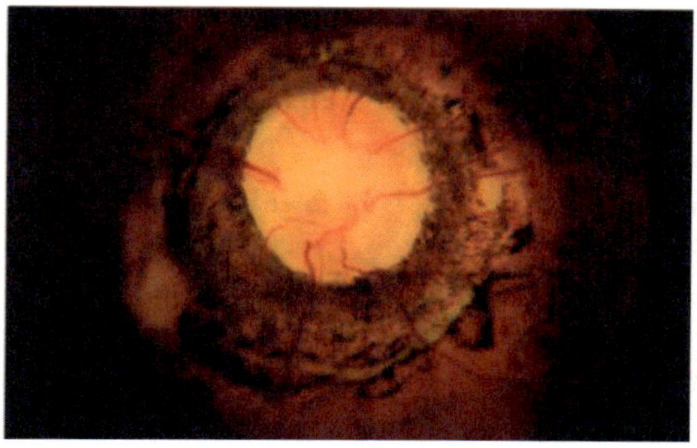

Figure 3. Morning glory syndrome.

usually occurs as an isolated ocular anomaly, or can also be associated with other ocular abnormalities such as strabismus, afferent pupillary defect, visual field defects, preretinal gliosis, and open angle glaucoma [22–25]. The optic nerve has been reported to present with characteristics of coloboma, hypoplasia, and morning glory anomaly, as an overlapping phenotypic profile that has been described in relation to *PAX6* mutations, which influences the phenotypes of optic nerve malformations [26].

3.3. Optic nerve choristoma

Choristoma is an uncommon congenital tumor where normal-looking tissue (epithelial, glandular, cartilaginous, osseous, smooth muscle, and fat) is present in an area where it should not be normally present. Most ocular choristomas are periocular but can also be rarely found as an intraocular choristoma involving the iris, ciliary body, choroid, and optic nerve head [27]. The largest series on optic nerve choristomas in the English literature was published in 1972 including 26 cases of optic nerve colobomas in enucleated eyes, and all cases were diagnosed to have associated heterotopic adipose and/or smooth muscle tissue on pathological examination. The age at enucleation ranged from 6 weeks to 70 years [28]. An interesting case presenting with mixed clinical features of optic nerve coloboma and morning glory—as previously described by others—has been reported by Mishra but unexpectedly had histopathological evidence of a choristoma [29, 30]. The authors commented that there is insufficient knowledge in the literature about the natural history and outcome of optic nerve choristoma, but their 15-year old girl has shown dramatic rapid deterioration of vision. They attributed this to the abnormal architecture of the colobomatous nerve that resulted in the patient's vulnerability to the critical growth of the choristomatous tissue during adolescence, on the top of the slow axonal loss from the choristoma, as evident by the pallor of the optic nerve head at the time of presentation [30].

3.4. Optic nerve coloboma

Ocular coloboma occurs in relation to the failure of the closure of the embryonic fissure that results from the evagination of the developing optic vesicle during embryogenesis and eye development. The fissure is located inferiorly and includes the optic stalk (future optic nerve) that connects the developing forebrain to the eye. The extent of the colobomatous defect depends on the location of the arrested closure of that fissure. Colobomas in the eye can be seen anteriorly involving the iris and ciliary body or posteriorly involving the optic nerve. The optic nerve coloboma appears as a sharp whitish excavation inferiorly with a thin neuroretinal rim and may even extend to involve the adjacent choroidal and retinal tissue. Optic disc colobomas can occur bilaterally, can be sporadic, or can have an autosomal dominant inheritance. Ocular coloboma is known to show extensive locus heterogeneity associated with causative mutations identified in genes encoding developmental transcription factors or components of signaling pathways that are involved in the posterior segment development as a whole. Optic nerve coloboma can be associated with similar colobomatous anterior uveal or posterior chorioretinal defect as well as possible more extensive manifestations (anophthalmia/microphthalmia) related to the defective and/or failure of embryonic fissure closure [30]. The term microphthalmia is used to indicate the marked reduction in the size of an eye. Microphthalmia, anophthalmia, and coloboma resulting from failure of optic fissure closure during embryogenesis have been grouped as a single phenotype or spectrum (MAC) in most of the recent studies aiming at identification of responsible genes [31, 32]. Heterozygous loss-of-function mutations in *SOX2*, *PAX6*, and *OTX2* (involving dosage-sensitive transcription factors) are the most common genetic pathology associated with severe eye malformations (anophthalmos/severe microphthalmos) [33–36], and bi-allelic loss-of- function in *STRA6*, *ALDH1A3*, and *RARB* (related to the regulation of retinoic acid metabolism or transport) is confirmed as an emerging cause of nonsyndromic eye malformations [37–40]. In the coloboma/microphthalmia patients, Prokudin reported other variants in CYP1B1 that are emerging with *CYP1B1* being considered a possible candidate gene as a modifier in coloboma/microphthalmia [41] and commented on the heterogeneity and the complex pattern associated with MAC phenotype. This is nicely summarized by Reis and Semina [32]. Two novel heterozygous *SOX11* variants were identified in patients with coloboma [42]. In general, an identifiable genetic cause is found by molecular genetic testing in 80% of individuals with bilateral anophthalmia/severe microphthalmia and in up to 20% of individuals with an ocular malformation in the MAC spectrum [43]. Microphthalmos is one of the ocular anomalies described in fetal alcohol syndrome, which causes multiple teratogenic effects on ocular embryogenesis [44]. Lenz microphthalmia syndrome (LMS) is a specific entity characterized by unilateral or bilateral microphthalmia and/or clinical anophthalmia with malformations of the ears, teeth, fingers, skeleton, and/or genitourinary system in addition to coloboma, which is present in 60% of microphthalmic eyes. The coloboma ranges from simple iris coloboma to coloboma of the ciliary body, choroid, and ON. The diagnosis of LMS depends on clinical findings; however, molecular testing showed that *NAA10* and *BCOR* (BCL6 corepressor) are known to be associated with LMS.

3.5. Optic nerve aplasia

Optic nerve (ON) aplasia is a rare developmental anomaly that implies complete absence of the ON including the disc and is usually seen in unilateral deformed globe in a healthy person with no hereditary predisposition. There are only three previous reports of bilateral ON aplasia in otherwise normal children [45–47]. The radiological finding of thinned ON indicates the presence of ON sheath with some glial tissue and can aid in the diagnosis. In the most recent case, flash visually evoked potentials (VEP) was performed to distinguish ON hypoplasia from ON aplasia and VEP was not recordable [47]. The ON is formed of axons of the retinal ganglion cells, which form the ON that is derived embryologically from the inner neuroblastic layer of the optic cup, and failure of development of these cells is rare [48]. When there is accompanying failure of development of mesodermal elements as well, it is termed aplasia of the ON, which is defined as an absence of optic nerve, ganglion cells, and central retinal vessels [28, 49]. Many previously reported cases in literature as ON aplasia are, actually, cases of ON hypoplasia because of some overlapping features [50]. Variable ophthalmic features associated with ON aplasia include microphthalmos, enophthalmos, ptotic lids, squint, microcornea, trabeculodysgenesis, iris hypoplasia, iris coloboma, aniridia, and persistent hyperplastic primary vitreous [28, 49].

3.6. Optic nerve hypoplasia (ONH)

Unilateral ONH is a congenital disorder characterized by an underdevelopment of one of the ONs with marked intracranial asymmetry. Clinically, the ON head looks small with a characteristic "double-ring sign" (**Figure 4**). Visual acuity ranges from 20/20 to amaurosis presenting variable visual field defects but the visual impairment is nonprogressive. The diagnosis of ONH is typically clinical, but the confirmation is more accurately established by MRI [51, 52]. Several associations have also been reported between ONH and central nervous system (CNS) anomalies: such as septo-optic dysplasia (SOD), which is a heterogeneous inconstant combination of different CNS parenchymal malformations: ONH, pituitary hypoplasia (with hormonal deficiency), and midline malformations of the brain (absence of the septum pellucidum or thinning of the corpus callosum) [52]. On the other hand, several anomalies have been reported in fetal alcohol syndrome including optic nerve hypoplasia in 48%, and abnormal tortuosity of retinal arteries in 49% in addition to anterior segment anomalies such as microcornea, cataract, and iris defects in 10% [53]. The ONH is thought to occur because of the teratogenic of alcohol on the developing optic nerve at sixth week of gestation when the first retinal ganglion cells first appear until after birth [44]. It is recommended to perform neuroimaging when ONH is

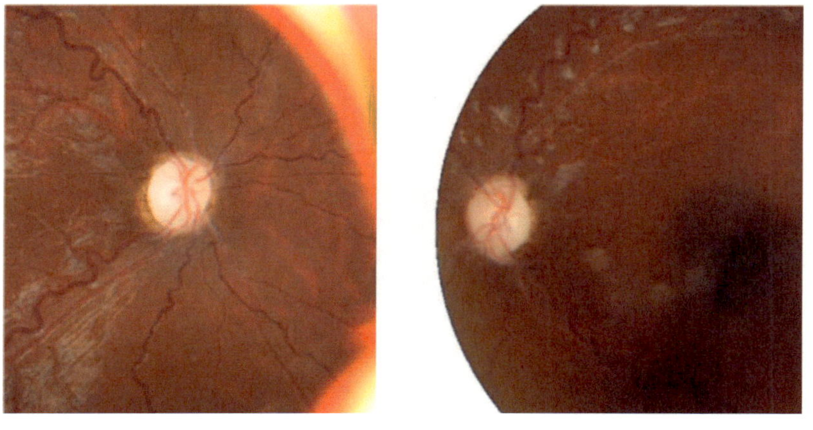

Figure 4. Bilateral optic nerve hypoplasia in a patient with septo-optic dysplasia.

detected to rule out other associated CNS anomalies and internal carotid artery hypoplasia, which has been recently reported advocating the theory of vascular disruption sequence at the time of neuroembryogenesis and restriction of intrauterine blood supply as the cause for ONH [54]. Patients with ONH should also have endocrinological work-up to rule out de Morsier syndrome since hypothalamic/pituitary dysfunction has been found in 69% of unilateral cases and 81% in bilateral [55, 56]. ONH has been reported in association with Down's syndrome in the United States [57]. Optic nerve dysplasia and vascular anomalies have also been found in 4–38% of patients with Down's syndrome in emerging countries [58, 59]. Afifi and co-authors also reported tilted (dysplastic) optic nerve heads in two cases out of their studied series of Down's syndrome children but related their finding to an associated myopia in the same two patients [60]. ONH is the most common congenital ON anomaly and a major cause of blindness in the USA, and even though most cases are isolated, the new molecular diagnostic techniques have recently raised the fact that a significant portion of ONH cases has underlying genetic causes, typically de novo mutations [61] Also, two missense mutations in SALL4 were found in a patient with bilateral ONH, unilateral microphthalmos, and coloboma, in addition to cardiac septal defects and delayed growth. *SALL4* is expressed in the developing lens and regulates BMP4; therefore, authors speculated that altered *BMP4* expression is the cause for the eye anomalies [62]. Finally, it has been suggested to perform behavioral assessment in ONH children who have mild to moderate or even no visual impairment [63].

3.7. Optic tract hypoplasia

Congenital optic tract hypoplasia is rare and most of the optic tract abnormalities are acquired [64]. They are usually attributed to tumor, hemorrhage, aneurism, and CNS demyelinating disease, while some are associated with anophthalmos. Isolated optic tract aplasia/hypoplasia was reported in three cases, all of which are unilateral [65–67].

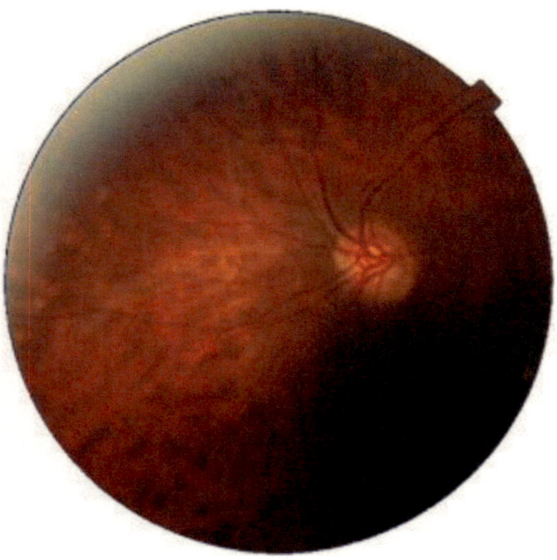

Figure 5. Tilted disc syndrome.

3.8. Optic nerve (ON) tilt

ON tilt has been described in association with myopia and more strongly in association with the presence of crescent regardless of the refractive error (**Figure 5**). Crescent was observed approximately five times more frequently in myopic eyes when compared with nonmyopic eyes (49 vs. 10%), and the median degree of tilt was about double (6.08 vs. 2.48). Ethnicity was also strongly associated with tilt and crescent, with ON heads in Asian eyes having the most tilt [68].

4. Primary tumors of the optic nerve

4.1. Optic pathway glioma (OPG or pilocytic astrocytoma)

Optic pathway gliomas (OPGs) comprise tumors that arise from the visual pathway including the optic nerve (ON) and chiasm. Tumors that only affect the ON are referred to as optic nerve gliomas (ONGs). In general, OPGs are uncommon and account for only about 1% of intracranial tumors [69]. However, they are the most common primary tumors of the optic nerve, comprising about 65% of all intrinsic ON tumors [70].

More than two-thirds of OPGs are detected in the first decade of life and up to 90% before the end of the second decade [69]. The median age of diagnosis of ONGs is 6.5 years with an age range of 2–46 years. Whereas the median age of chiasmal gliomas is 11 years with an age range of 0.75–50 years [71]. There is no sex predilection. Those lesions are considered hamartomas by some authors. ONGs are considered by the 2016 World Health Organization (WHO) as low-grade I juvenile pilocytic astrocytomas or grade II diffuse fibrillary astrocytomas [72].

ONGs are most often benign and slowly growing. The most common presenting findings in descending order are proptosis (94%), vision loss (87.5%), optic disc pallor (59%), disc edema (35%), and strabismus (27%) [69]. However, the presentation of ONGs is variable and mostly depends on the segment of the optic nerve affected by the tumor. The "anterior" involvement presents with signs of an anterior optic neuropathy and is more likely to be associated with optic disc swelling. The "posterior" involvement is associated with either normal or pale optic disc. Patients infrequently present with isolated optic atrophy. A relative afferent pupillary defect (RAPD) is usually present in unilateral or asymmetric cases with affected visual field. The occurrence of nystagmus represents severe visual loss. The nystagmus is monocular, vertical, of low-frequency and variable amplitude. This can differentiate it from spasmus nutans, which is known to be seen in gliomas that involve the optic chiasm [73]. Other rare presentations of ONGs include central retinal vein occlusion (CRVO), retinochoroidal collaterals, or neovascular glaucoma (NVG) [74].

Most cases of ONGs are sporadic. However, there is a clear genetic relationship between ONGs and neurofibromatosis type 1 (NF1). NF1 is an autosomal dominant disorder that occurs in 1 in 3000 individuals. It is caused by a mutation in the gene coding for neurofibromin, a tumor suppressor gene, situated in chromosome 17. About 8–31% of NF1 patients have ONGs. On the other hand, 10–70% of patients with ONGs have NF1 [75]. The wide range of incidence can be explained by referral bias, radiologic detection rate, and the used diagnostic criteria.

The etio-pathogenesis for the development of gliomas in patients with NF1 is related to the activation of the retro-virus-associated sequence (RAS) oncogene (that is inhibited by neurofibromin in normal individuals) and the B1 homolog of the retrovirus-associated function (BRAF) oncogene [73]. The end result is increased protein synthesis and glial cell proliferation. The association between NF1 and the behavior of the glioma is poorly understood. Classically, optic nerve gliomas in patients with NF1 have a more benign prognosis, although this concern is unresolved [69]. Rarely, ONGs can be found in patients with neurofibromatosis type 2 (NF2) [76]. In addition, ipsilateral optic nerve glioma can occur in association with morning glory disc anomaly [77].

Regarding the radiologic findings (**Figure 6**), ONGs may show one of two patterns. The most common pattern is the classic fusiform swelling of the ON. In magnetic resonance imaging (MRI), they are hypo- or isointense in T1-weighted images, hyperintense in T2-weighted images, enhancing after intravenous injection gadolinium. The subarachnoid space (SAS) surrounding the ONGs is distended and thought to be occupied by trapped cerebrospinal fluid (CSF) in some patients. However, ultrasonographic examination in such cases characteristically discloses signs of solid component in the SAS. This indicates that the distension is most likely due to the spread of tumor into the SAS (the "pseudo-CSF sign") and does not represent trapped CSF [78].

The second and less common radiologic pattern is the appearance of a thickened and kinked nerve in the portion affected by the ONG [75, 76]. Like the first pattern, enlargement of the subarachnoid space is due to extension of the tumor. It was suggested that this pattern (i.e., thickening and kinking) is more commonly observed in patients with NF1 and the fusiform enlargement pattern is more commonly seen in patients with sporadic ONG [79]. Nevertheless, no pattern is indicative of a specific diagnosis as both can be seen in sporadic ONGs and ONGs related to NF1. In both patterns, the margin of the nerve is usually well defined and smooth due to an intact optic nerve sheath. This is a differentiating feature between ONG and optic nerve sheath meningioma (ONSM).

ONGs can either show an isolated involvement of the orbital portion of the optic nerve or combined involvement of both orbital and intracranial portions. The optic foramen may still be distended even if the ONG is restricted to the orbital or intracranial portion of the optic

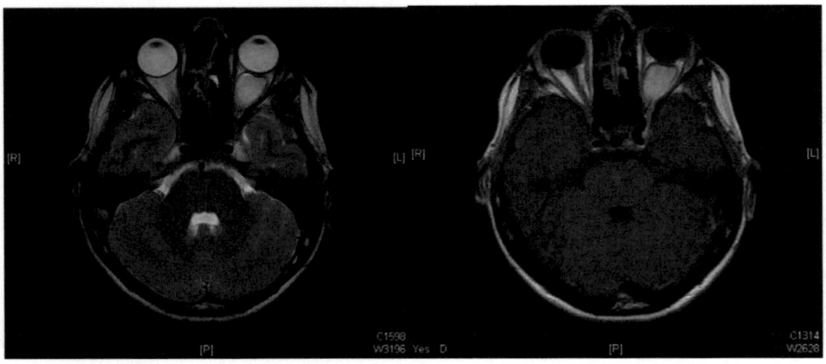

Figure 6. Optic nerve glioma. The left figure is a T2-weighted axial MRI showing left orbital and intraconal mass with high signal intensity. The right figure is a T1-weighted axial MRI showing postcontrast enhancement.

nerve. This is caused by secondary meningeal hyperplasia traveling proximally (or distally) and not the tumor itself. Therefore, enlargement of the optic foramen is not a proof of intracranial extension of an orbital ONG. Furthermore, the optic foramen may still be of normal diameter in the sitting of intracranial or chiasmal ONG [80]. Histopathologic examination performed on a resected ONG, which did not reveal spread intracranially by MRI as well as by gross examination, showed an evidence of intracranial spread [81].

Histopathologically (**Figure 7**), ONGs are characterized by three main patterns that may all be present in different cuts of the same tumor: **A.** Transitional area, in which the tumor blends into the normal tissue of optic nerve and shows more abundant and less arranged glial nuclei than in the normal nerve. Increased number and size of glial cells results in enlarged nerve bundles. **B.** Coarsely reticulated and myxomatous areas with microcystoid spaces perhaps representing tumor necrosis. **C.** Astrocytic areas, in which spindle cell formation with Rosenthal fibers, which are cytoplasmic and eosinophilic structures in astrocytes, are seen [80]. Immunohistochemically, the neoplastic astrocytes stain positively for glial fibrillary acidic protein, HNK-1 (type 1 astrocyte precursor marker), S-100, and vimentin. Thus, this suggests that type 1 astrocytes are the origin of the tumor [82]. ONGs nearly always remain confined to the dural sheath, but a spread into the subarachnoid space surrounding the nerve is not uncommon [75].

The diagnosis of an ONG is usually reached on the basis of the clinical signs and radiologic findings. Biopsy of the lesion is largely not required because of the presence of high-resolution neuroimaging with enhanced diagnostic accuracy, biopsy of the sheath alone may show secondary meningeal hyperplasia seen in ONGs and falsely suggesting optic nerve sheath meningioma, and the low predictive value of the histologic appearance of the tumor in its clinical behavior [82]. Most importantly, the procedure could be complicated by permanent visual loss [83].

There is no universally recognized management for ONGs, and it should be individualized to the patient. ONGs are usually very slow growing tumors and some lesions will spontaneously regress. Therefore, observation is indicated for patients with reasonably good vision

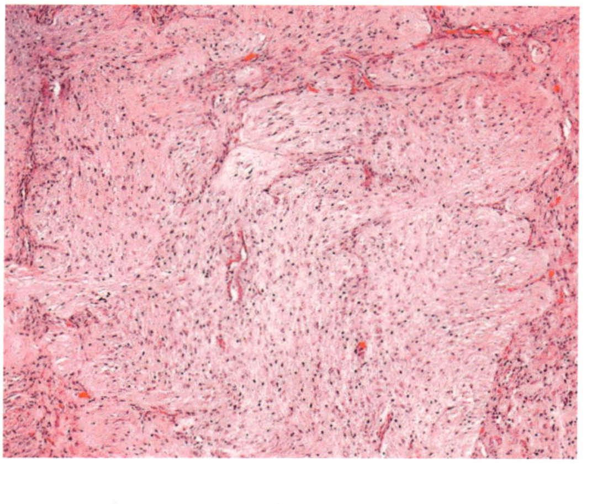

Figure 7. Histopathological appearance of an optic nerve pilocytic astrocytoma (Original magnification × 100 hematoxylin and eosin).

and stable radiologic appearance on serial imaging [84, 85]. For patients presenting with reduced vision and particularly if it is deteriorating or there is a radiologic evidence of tumor growth, a number of treatment options exists.

Chemotherapy is evolving as an initial treatment modality for patients with severe or progressive visual deterioration. It may be especially beneficial in children younger than 5 years of age. The recommended chemotherapeutic agents include vincristine, carboplatin, vinblastine, and temozolomide with remarkable outcomes observed in some patients [86]. Combining carboplatin and vincristine is the most accepted regimen [69]. Additionally, treatment with topical nerve growth factor improved the vision in patients with known or presumed ONGs. A 10-day course of topical murine nerve growth factor in five children with ONGs and severe optic disc pallor showed an increase in visual evoked potential amplitudes that lasted for 90 days in all patients [87].

Fractionated stereotactic radiotherapy is another option for some patients with ONGs and can be used as a monotherapy or adjunctive to other treatment modalities [88, 89]. It is usually kept for patients who are older than 5 years of age and, preferably, after puberty. Shrinkage of ONGs, with subsequent improvement in vision and halting of progressive visual loss, reduction in optic disc swelling, and decreasing proptosis have been reported in two studies [90, 91]. In contrast, a third study concluded that radiation of ONGs has no significant benefit in the overall outcome when compared to observation or surgical intervention [71]. Thus, radiotherapy is still controversial because of questionable results and possible complications including pituitary dysfunction and intellectual disabilities [69].

Surgical excision or debulking of ONGs may be indicated in patients with severe deterioration of visual function associated with cosmetically disfiguring proptosis [92, 93]. In some cases, optic nerve sheath fenestration is performed to release the trapped CSF surrounding the tumor. Surgery has been suggested to prevent progression into the intracranial optic nerve and chiasm. However, involvement of the chiasm is rare and prevention is not proven as the tumor was commonly found in the margins during histopathologic examination of the resected ONGs [82].

4.2. Malignant optic nerve glioma (malignant astrocytoma)

Malignant ONGs are rare neoplasms that involve the anterior visual pathway (i.e., proximal to the lateral geniculate nucleus). According to the WHO 2016, malignant ONGs are classified as grade III (anaplastic astrocytoma) or grade IV (glioblastoma) [72]. In contrast to ONGs mentioned above, malignant ONGs predominantly affects adults. The mean age of onset is 57 years with an age range between 22 and 83 years. There is no gender predilection [94]. Patients present acutely with unilateral or bilateral orbital pain and progressive vision loss. The optic disc appearance can be either normal or pale in most cases although disc swelling and CRVO can also occur [75, 94].

MRI scan shows diffusely enlarged optic nerve, chiasm, or optic tract with heterogenous enhancement [69]. Histopathologically, malignant ONGs are show areas of anaplasia and are classified as anaplastic astrocytomas or glioblastoma multiforme [78]. Treatment involves radiotherapy, chemotherapy, or both but is rarely successful. The visual and the survival rate are very poor. Blindness typically occurs 2 to 4 months after onset of vision loss and mortality from hypothalamic and brainstem involvement usually follows after 6–12 months [69].

4.3. ON medulloepithelioma

Medulloepithelioma refers to tumors arising from the cells of the primitive neural tube and the medullary plate. These tumors are extremely rare [95]. They can arise in any part of the central or peripheral nervous system [96, 97]. They may also arise from the globe, principally the ciliary body. Medulloepitheliomas arising from the optic nerve are very rare. Patients present with proptosis, progressive visual loss, disc swelling, and later disc pallor [73].

Imaging initially may show fusiform enlargement of the ON resembling an ONG [75]. At the time of surgery, the diagnosis of an ON medulloepithelioma is usually reached. Histopathologic examination of ON Medulloepithelioma shows hyperchromatic nuclei with high mitotic index. The neoplastic cells are arranged in tubes and cords. Hyaluronidase-sensitive material is observed and stains positively with Alcian blue [75, 98, 99]. More differentiated cells are arranged in rosettes [73]. Teratoid variants of medulloepithelioma have other elements such as striated muscle or cartilage [78, 98].

The most commonly used treatment modality is resection of the involved ON. Even with complete resection, however, recurrences and metastases can be seen. Therefore, other treatment options include adjuvant radiotherapy, chemotherapy, or both [75, 99].

4.4. ON oligodendroglioma

Oligodendroglioma is a type of glioma that is believed to originate from oligodendrocytes. Up to 12% of all intracranial tumors are caused by oligodendrogliomas [100], and there is no gender predilection. They can affect individuals on all ages although they are more prevalent in middle aged adults. The most common location of oligodendrogliomas is in the cerebral hemispheres, particularly the frontal lobes. However, oligodendrogliomas of the cerebellum, the spinal cord, and the brainstem have been reported [101].

Histopathologically, compact masses of swollen oligodendrocytes were separated by an extremely thin stroma. Mitoses are generally rare and variable [100]. They have been reported to be associated with orbital non-Hodgkin lymphoma [102]. Another study described a case of a 14-year-old girl who presented with monocular progressive proptosis, vision loss, and limited extraocular muscle motility. Imaging showed a large fusiform enlargement of the orbital portion of the ON. Microscopic examination of the resected ON proved changes indicative of an oligodendroglioma [103].

4.5. ON ganglioglioma

As the name implies, gangliogliomas are composed of both ganglion cells and astrocytes. They are rare tumors and classified as grade I by the WHO [72]. Gangliogliomas of the ON have been described in few studies [104–106]. In noncontrast enhanced imaging, ON ganglioglioma resembles a benign ONG. However, gangliogliomas characteristically do not show enhancement on MRI after intravenous injection of gadolinium [104]. However, the diagnosis of ON gangliogliomas is usually reached after microscopic examination that shows many ganglion cells with an increased population of glial cells. Treatment involves partial or total ON nerve resection and radiotherapy [73].

4.6. ON hemangioblastoma

ON hemangioblastomas may be sporadic or occur in the sitting of Von Hippel-Lindau disease (VHL). It is an extremely rare tumor, which affects males and females equally with an age of onset ranging from 15 to 44 years. Presentation includes vision loss, headaches or pain with ocular movement, and proptosis accompanied by optic disc swelling or pallor [107]. Radiologically, they look like ONGs except that hemangioblastomas show more homogenous enhancement. Histopathologically, these tumors are comprised of endothelial cells and pericytes with variably sized vascular channels [73].

4.7. ON schwannoma

Schwannomas are benign tumors of peripheral nervous systems derived from Schwann cells. The vestibular location of the schwannoma is more frequent, followed by the involvement of the trigeminal nerve. In the orbit, schwannomas account for 1–6% of intraorbital tumors. Although it is theoretically impossible for a schwannoma to develop from the sheath of the optic nerve, which is devoid of Schwann cells, there are some exceptional cases of schwannoma of the nerve [108–111].

Several histopathogenic explanations have been reported. These include the presence of ectopic Schwann cells that may have migrated at the time of embryogenesis [110, 112]. Another explanation would be a transformation of the pial mesenchymal cells [112, 113]. A final hypothesis is that schwannoma does not develop from the sheath of the optic nerve but from sympathetic nerves running on it [75, 110]. T1-weighted MRI typically demonstrates a homogenously enhancing lesion. The complete excision of these tumors most often allows a definitive cure without recurrence [114, 115].

5. Primary tumors of the optic nerve sheath (optic nerve sheath meningioma)

The only tumor that can develop solely from the optic nerve sheath is optic nerve sheath meningioma (ONSM) [73]. ONSMs result from proliferations of the meningoepithelial cells covering the sheath of the intraorbital or intracanalicular optic nerve [69]. ONSMs are uncommon, accounting for 1–2% of all orbital tumors [116–118]. However, ONSMs are the second most common cause of primary optic nerve and sheath tumors, second only to optic nerve glioma [69]. Moreover, 90% of all orbital meningiomas were secondary to intracranial extension and the remaining 10% were primary ONSMs [116].

Almost all ONSMs are unilateral although they may be bilateral especially in patients with NF2 [119]. ONSMs are typically discovered in adults during the fourth or fifth decade. Females are affected three times as often as males. Up to 7% of all ONSMs occur in children [69]. A classification system of ONSMs was suggested and includes three types: type I ONSMs, in which the tumor involves the orbital portion of the ON manifesting as fusiform, tubular, or globular enlargement of the nerve; type II ONSMs, where the tumor extends through the optic canal or supraorbital fissure; and type III ONSMs, with more than 10-mm intracranial extension or involvement of the contralateral ON [120].

The classic diagnostic triad of ONSMs includes painless, slowly progressive, unilateral vision loss associated with optic atrophy, and retinochoroidal collaterals. These collateral vessels connect the retinal venous circulation to the choroidal venous circulation and are seen in approximately 30% of patients [69]. Transient visual obscuration may also occur. In addition, reduced color vision, visual field defect, an ipsilateral RAPD with variable proptosis and limitation of ocular motility are observed [73]. The ON head maybe normal, swollen, or atrophic, depending on duration of symptoms and the location of the tumor [75, 116–118].

Radiological findings of ONSMs are variable (**Figure 8**). Computed tomography (CT) scanning characteristically shows fusiform or tubular expansion of the affected with a thickened and enhanced optic nerve sheath. Calcification of the sheath gives the classic "tram-track" sign. MRI is more accurate in soft tissue definition and proves that the ON parenchyma is of normal diameter. The ON is hypointense in T1-weighted images with the optic nerve sheath showing increased thickness and marked enhancement. In contrast to ONGs that show a smooth dural outline, ONSMs show rough outlines with thin extensions from the affected sheath [116–118].

Histopathologically (**Figures 9 and 10**), ONSMs have a meningotheliomatous or a mixed-type pattern. Psammoma bodies, which are hyalinized calcium deposits, are usually seen. Commonly, meningiomas spread to the extradural space invading the orbital tissue. Rarely, optic nerve, sclera, choroid, and retina are invaded [73, 80]. The diagnosis of ONSM primarily depends on the clinical presentation and imaging without the need for a biopsy in most cases [72].

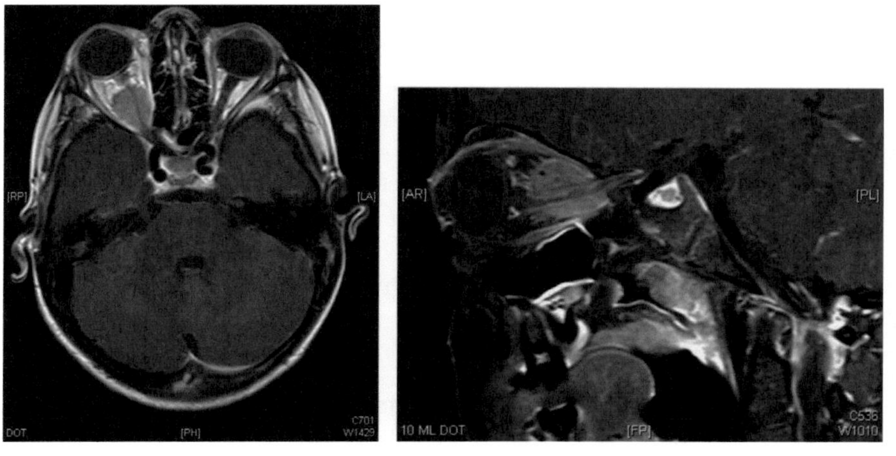

Figure 8. Optic nerve sheath meningioma. T1-weighted MRI showing right oval orbital space occupying lesion encasing the mid and posterior right optic nerve.

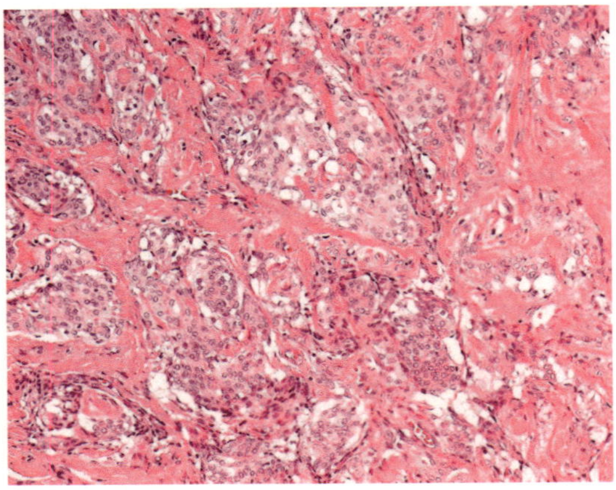

Figure 9. The histopathological appearance of the whorl-configuration of meningothelial cell proliferation (original magnification × 200 hematoxylin and eosin).

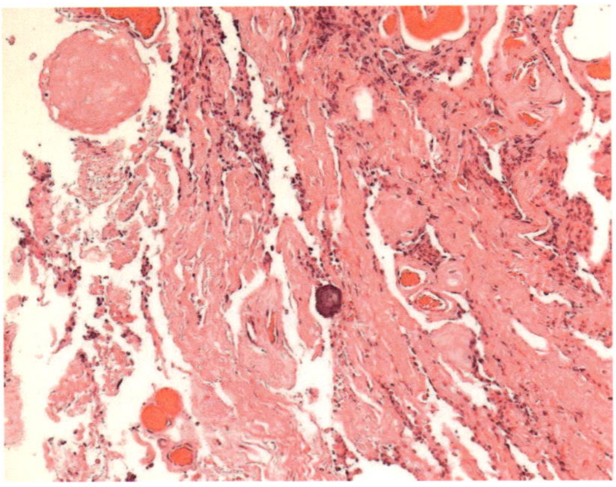

Figure 10. The appearance of the typical psammoma bodies in the same case of the optic nerve meningioma above (original magnification × 200 hematoxylin and eosin).

The only ONSMs related morbidity is visual loss from injury to the ipsilateral ON. These tumors typically do not cause neurological dysfunction or death. Therefore, the management of patients with ONSMs should be tailored to the individual case. Observation is suitable if there is no significant visual loss at presentation or follow-up, and there is no significant intracranial extension. Those patients can be observed twice per year with serial imaging [73]. ONSMs in pediatric population maybe more aggressive, and thus, they must be monitored with increased frequency [69].

Fractionated radiation therapy is the mainstay treatment of ONSM. More than 94% of patients' vision has stabilized or improved. However, late radiation complications include radiation retinopathy and pituitary dysfunction [73]. Surgical excision is rarely advised because of the potential risk of significant visual deterioration. Indications for surgical intervention include intracranial extension of the tumor if there is a risk of contralateral ON involvement [69, 121].

6. Secondary tumors of the optic nerve and sheath

Secondary tumors of the optic nerve are more common than the primary tumors [122]. These tumors can damage the ON by either infiltration, compression, or both. Secondary tumors include retinoblastoma, malignant melanoma of choroid, pseudotumor of the RPE, intracranial meningioma, metastatic carcinoma to the ON parenchyma or ONS, glioblastoma multiforme of the brain, lymphoma, or leukemia [73]. The clinical signs and management of secondary tumors depend on the particular tumor and the location of damage to the ON.

Conflict of interest

We do not have any financial interests in any of the listed items in this manuscript.

Author details

Hind Alkatan*, Daniah Alshowaeir and Tariq Alzahem

*Address all correspondence to: hindkatan@yahoo.com

King Saud University, Riyadh, Kingdom of Saudi Arabia

References

[1] Miller NR, Walsh FB, Hoyt WF. Walsh and Hoyt's Clinical Neuro-Ophthalmology. Pennsylvania, United States: Lippincott Williams & Wilkins; 2005

[2] Zhang J, Rubin R, Rao N. Anatomy and Embryology of the Optic Nerve: Duane's Foundations of Clinical Ophthalmology. Philadelphia: Lippincott Williams & Wilkins; 2005. pp. 1-10

[3] Mikelberg FS, Drance SM, Schulzer M, Yidegiligne HM, Weis MM. The normal human optic nerve: Axon count and axon diameter distribution. Ophthalmology. 1989;**96**(9):1325-1328

[4] Remington LA. Clinical Anatomy of the Visual System. Butterworths-Heinemann. Oxford, United Kingdom: Elsevier Health Sciences; 2011

[5] Adler FH, Kaufman PL, Levin LA, Alm A. Adler's Physiology of the Eye. Saunders. Philadelphia, United States: Elsevier Health Sciences. 2011

[6] Adrian ED, Matthews BHC. The Berger rhythm: Potential changes from the occipital lobes in man. Brain. 1934;**57**:355-385

[7] Ciganek L. The EEG response (evoked potential) to light stimulus in man. Electroencephalography and Clinical Neurophysiology. 1961;**13**(2):165-172

[8] Halliday A, McDonald W, Mushin J. Delayed visual evoked response in optic neuritis. Lancet. 1972;**299**(7758):982-985

[9] Hoffmann MB, Seufert PS, Bach M. Simulated nystagmus suppresses pattern-reversal but not pattern-onset visual evoked potentials. Clinical Neurophysiology. 2004;**115**(11): 2659-2665

[10] Saunders KJ, Brown G, McCulloch DL. Pattern-onset visual evoked potentials: More useful than reversal for patients with nystagmus. Documenta Ophthalmologica. 1997;**94**(3):265-274

[11] Odom JV, Bach M, Brigell M, Holder GE, McCulloch DL, Tormene AP. ISCEV standard for clinical visual evoked potentials (2009 update). Documenta Ophthalmologica. 2010;**120**(1):111-119

[12] Heckenlively JR, John R, Arden GB, editors. Principles and Practice of Clinical Electrophysiology of Vision. Cambridge, Massachusetts, United States: MIT Press; 2006

[13] Straatsma BR, Foos BY, Heckenlively JR, Taylor GN. Myelinated retinal nerve fibers. American Journal of Ophthalmology. 1981;**91**:25-38

[14] Shelton JB, Digre KB, Gilman J, Warner JE, Katz BJ. Characteristics of myelinated retinal nerve fiber layer in ophthalmic imaging: Findings on autofluorescence, fluorescein angiographic, infrared, optical coherence tomographic, and red-free images. JAMA Ophthalmology. 2013;**131**(1):107e109

[15] Walsh DM, Merson TD, Landman KA, Hughes BD1. Evidence for cooperative selection of axons for myelination by adjacent oligodendrocytes in the optic nerve. PLoS One. 2016;**11**(11):e0165673. DOI: 10.1371/journal.pone.0165673. eCollection 2016

[16] Garcia GA, Tian JJ, Apinyawasisuk S, Kim S, Aki H, Sadun AA. Clues from Crouzon: Insights into the potential role of growth factors in the pathogenesis of myelinated retinal nerve fibers. Journal of Current Ophthalmology. 2016;**28**:232e236. http://www.journals.elsevier.com/journal-of-current-ophthalmology

[17] Pendler C. Unusual coloboma of the optic nerve entrance. The British Journal of Ophthalmology. 1961;**45**:803-807

[18] Kindler P. Morning glory syndrome: Unusual congenital optic disc anomaly. American Journal of Ophthalmology. 1970;**69**:376-384

[19] Ribeiro-da-Silva J. Congenital optic disc deformities. A clinical approach. Ophthalmic Paediatrics and Genetics. 1985;**5**(1-2):67-70

[20] Brodsky MC. Congenital optic disk anomalies. Survey of Ophthalmology. 1994;**39**:89-112

[21] Steinkuller PG. The morning glory disk anomaly: Case report and literature review. Journal of Pediatric Ophthalmology and Strabismus. 1980;**17**:81-87

[22] Jackson W, Freed S. Ocular and systemic abnormalities associated with morning glory syndrome. Ophthalmic Paediatrics and Genetics. 1985;**5**:111-115

[23] Jacobs M, Taylor D. The systemic and genetic significance of congenital optic disc anomalies. Eye. 1991;**5**:470-475

[24] Manschot W. Morning glory syndrome: A histopathological study. The British Journal of Ophthalmology. 1990;**74**:56-58

[25] Marija B, Paraskeva H-S, Vujica M, Ivan M. Morning glory syndrome associated with primary open angle glaucoma: Case report. Srpski Arhiv za Celokupno Lekarstvo. 2014;**142**(3-4):223-225. DOI: 10.2298/SARH1404223B

[26] Azuma N, Yamaguchi Y, Handa H, Tadokoro K, Asaka A, Kawasi E, Yamada M. Mutations of the *PAX6* gene detected in patients with a variety of optic-nerve malformations. American Journal of Human Genetics. 2003;**72**:1565-1570

[27] Kim BH, Henderson BA. Intraocular choristoma. Seminars in Ophthalmology. 2005; **20**(4):223-229

[28] Willis F, Zimmerman LE, O'Grady R, Smith RS, Crawford B. Heterotopic adipose tissue and smooth muscle in the optic disc: Association with isolated colobomas. Archives of Ophthalmology. 1972;**88**:139-146

[29] Brodsky M. Congenital optic disc anomalies. In: Hoyt C, Taylor D, editors. Pediatric Ophthalmology and Strabismus. London: Elsevier; 2013. pp. 543-560

[30] Mishra A, Heathcote JG, LaRoche GR. Optic nerve choristoma causing vision loss in an adolescent. Canadian Journal of Ophthalmology. 2017;**52**(4):e138-e140. DOI: 10.1016/j.jcjo.2016.12.004

[31] Berk AT1, Yaman A, Saatçi AO. Ocular and systemic findings associated with optic disc colobomas. Journal of Pediatric Ophthalmology and Strabismus. 2003;**40**(5):272-278

[32] Skalicky SE, White AJ, Grigg JR, Martin F. Microphthalmia, anophthalmia, and coloboma and associated ocular and systemic features: Understanding the spectrum. JAMA Ophthalmology. 2013;**131**(12):1517-1524. DOI: 10.1001/jamaophthalmol.2013.5305

[33] Reis LM, Semina EV. Conserved genetic pathways associated with microphthalmia, anophthalmia, and coloboma. Birth Defects Research. Part C, Embryo Today. 2015;**105**(2): 96-113. DOI: 10.1002/bdrc.21097. Epub 2015 Jun 3

[34] Fantes J, Ragge NK, Lynch SA, McGill NI, Collin JR, Howard-Peebles PN, Hayward C, Vivian AJ, Williamson K, van Heyningen V, FitzPatrick DR. Mutations in SOX2 cause anophthalmia. Nature Genetics. 2003;**33**:461-463

[35] Ragge NK, Lorenz B, Schneider A, Bushby K, de Sanctis L, de Sanctis U, Salt A, Collin JR, Vivian AJ, Free SL, et al. SOX2 anophthalmia syndrome. American Journal of Medical Genetics. Part A. 2005;**135**:1-7. Discussion 8

[36] Ragge NK, Brown AG, Poloschek CM, Lorenz B, Henderson RA, Clarke MP, Russell-Eggitt I, Fielder A, Gerrelli D, Martinez-Barbera JP, et al. Heterozygous mutations of OTX2 cause severe ocular malformations. American Journal of Human Genetics. 2005;**76**:1008-1022

[37] Glaser T, Jepeal L, Edwards JG, Young SR, Favor J, Maas RL. PAX6 gene dosage effect in a family with congenital cataracts, aniridia, anophthalmia and central nervous system defects. Nature Genetics. 1994;**7**:463-471

[38] Pasutto F, Sticht H, Hammersen G, Gillessen-Kaesbach G, Fitzpatrick DR, Nurnberg G, Brasch F, Schirmer-Zimmermann H, Tolmie JL, Chitayat D, et al. Mutations in STRA6 cause a broad spectrum of malformations including anophthalmia, congenital heart defects, diaphragmatic hernia, alveolar capillary dysplasia, lung hypoplasia, and mental retardation. American Journal of Human Genetics. 2007;**80**:550-560

[39] Fares-Taie L, Gerber S, Chassaing N, Clayton-Smith J, Hanein S, Silva E, Serey M, Serre V, Ge´rard X, Baumann C, et al. ALDH1A3 mutations cause recessive anophthalmia and microphthalmia. American Journal of Human Genetics. 2013;**92**:265-270

[40] Srour M, Chitayat D, Caron V, Chassaing N, Bitoun P, Patry L, Cordier MP, Capo-Chichi JM, Francannet C, Calvas P, et al. Recessive and dominant mutations in retinoic acid receptor beta in cases with microphthalmia and diaphragmatic hernia. American Journal of Human Genetics. 2013;**93**:765-772

[41] Gerth-Kahlert C, Williamson K, Ansari M, Rainger JK, Hingst V, Zimmermann T, Tech S, Guthoff RF, van Heyningen V, FitzPatrick DR. Clinical and mutation analysis of 51 probands with anophthalmia and/or severe microphthalmia from a single center. Molecular Genetics & Genomic Medicine. 2013;**1**:15-31. DOI: 10.1002/mgg3.2

[42] Prokudin I, Simons C, Grigg JR, Storen R, Kumar V, Phua ZY, Smith J, Flaherty M, Davila S, Jamieson RV. Exome sequencing in developmental eye disease leads to identification of causal variants in GJA8, CRYGC, PAX6 and CYP1B1. European Journal of Human Genetics. 2014;**22**(7):907-915. DOI: 10.1038/ejhg.2013.268. Epub 2013 Nov 27

[43] Pillai-Kastoori L, Wen W, Wilson SG, Strachan E, Lo-Castro A, Fichera M, Musumeci SA, Lehmann OJ, Morris AC. Sox11 is required to maintain proper levels of Hedgehog signaling during vertebrate ocular morphogenesis. PLoS Genetics. 2014;**10**(7):e1004491. DOI: 10.1371/journal.pgen.1004491. eCollection 2014 Jul

[44] Bardakjian T, Weiss A, Schneider A. Microphthalmia/anophthalmia/coloboma spectrum. In: Pagon RA, Adam MP, Ardinger HH, Wallace SE, Amemiya A, LJH B, Bird TD, Ledbetter N, Mefford HC, RJH S, Stephens K, editors. Gene Reviews [Internet]. Seattle, WA: University of Washington; 1993-2017. 2004 Jan 29 [Updated 2015 Jul 9]

[45] Chan T, Bowell R, O'Keefe M, Lanigan B. Ocular manifestations in fetal alcohol syndrome. British Journal of Ophthalmology. 1991;**75**:524-552

[46] Scott IU, Warman R, Altman N. Bilateral aplasia of the optic nerves, chiasm, and tracts in an otherwise healthy infant. American Journal of Ophthalmology. 1997;**124**:409-410. [PubMed: 9439374]

[47] Sanjari MS, Ghasemi Falavarjani K, Parvaresh MM, Kharazi HH, Kashkooli MB. Bilateral aplasia of the optic nerve, chiasm, and tracts in an otherwise healthy infant. British Journal of Ophthalmology. 2006;**90**:513-514. [PMCID: PMC1857006] [PubMed: 16547339]

[48] Khandgave TP, Kulkarni VN, Muzumdar DV, Puthran N. Bilateral optic nerve aplasia: A rare isolated central nervous system anomaly. Middle East African Journal of Ophthalmology. 2014;**21**(3):262-264. DOI: 10.4103/0974-9233.134690

[49] Nathalie F, Davis EA. Embryology of the eye. In: Yanoff M, Duker JS, editors. Ophthalmology. 2nd ed. Vol. 1. New Delhi: Elsevier; 2006. p. 24

[50] Brodsky MC. Anomalies of the optic disc. In: Miller NR, Newman NJ, editors. Walsh and Hoyt Clinical Neuro Ophthalmology. 5th ed. Vol. 1. Baltimore: Williams and Wilkins; 1998. pp. 799-800

[51] Alqahtani J. Optic nerve aplasia: A case report and literature review. Journal of Pediatric Neurosciences. 2008;**2**:150-153

[52] Lenhart PD, Desai NK, Bruce BB, Hutchinson AK, Lambert SR. The role of magnetic resonance imaging in diagnosing optic nerve hypoplasia. American Journal of Ophthalmology. 2014;**158**:1164-1171

[53] Brodsky MC. Pediatric Neuroophthalmology. 3rd ed. New York: Springer; 2016

[54] Strömland K, Ventura LO, Mirzaei L, Fontes de Oliveira K, Marcelino Bandim J, Parente Ivo A, Brandt C. Fetal alcohol spectrum disorders among children in a Brazilian orphanage. Birth Defects Research. Part A, Clinical and Molecular Teratology. 2015;**103**(3):178-185. DOI: 10.1002/bdra.23326. Epub 2014 Nov 5. PMID: 25371388

[55] Garcia-Medina JJ, del-Rio-Vellosillo M, Fares-Valdivia J, Alemañ-Romero L, Zanon-Moreno V, Pinazo-Duran MD. Optic nerve hypoplasia and internal carotid artery hypoplasia: A new association. Canadian Journal of Ophthalmology. Oct 2017;**52**(5):e173-e177. DOI: 10.1016/j.jcjo.2017.05.006

[56] Patel L, McNally RJ, Harrison E, et al. Geographical distribution of optic nerve hypoplasia and septo-optic dysplasia in Northwest England. The Journal of Pediatrics. 2006;**148**:85-88

[57] Harvey JP. Incidental bilateral optic nerve hypoplasia. BMJ Case Reports. 2017;**2017**:pii: bcr-2017-220343. DOI: 10.1136/bcr-2017-220343

[58] Awan KJ. Uncommon ocular changes in Down's syndrome (Mongolism). Journal of Pediatric Ophthalmology. 1977;**14**(4):215-216

[59] Berk AT, Saatci AO, Erçal MD, Tunç M, Ergin M. Ocular findings in 55 patients with Down's syndrome. Ophthalmic Genetics. 1996;**17**(1):15-19

[60] Ebeigbe JA, Akpalaba R. Ocular health status of subjects with Down's syndrome in Benin City, Nigeria. African Journal of Medicine and Medical Sciences. 2006;**35**(3):365-368

[61] Afifi HH, Abdel Azeem AA, El-Bassyouni HT, Gheith ME, Rizk A, Bateman JB. Distinct ocular expression in infants and children with down syndrome in Cairo, Egypt: Myopia and heart disease. JAMA Ophthalmology. 2013;**131**(8):1057-1066. DOI: 10.1001/jamaophthalmol.2013.644

[62] Chen CA, Yin J, Lewis RA, Schaaf CP. Genetic causes of optic nerve hypoplasia. Journal of Medical Genetics. 2017;**54**(7):441-449. DOI: 10.1136/jmedgenet-2017-104626. Epub 2017 May 1

[63] Ullah E, Wu D, Madireddy L, Lao R, Ling-Fung Tang P, Wan EB, Kopinsky S, Kwok PY, Schneider A, Baranzini S, Ansar M, Slavotinek A. Two missense mutations in SALL4 in a patient with microphthalmia, coloboma, and optic nerve hypoplasia. Ophthalmic Genetics. 2016;**23**:1-5

[64] Webb EA, O'Reilly MA, Clayden JD, Seunarine KK, Dale N, Salt A, Clark CA, Dattani MT. Reduced ventral cingulum integrity and increased behavioral problems in children with isolated optic nerve hypoplasia and mild to moderate or no visual impairment. PLoS One. 2013;**8**(3):e59048. DOI: 10.1371/journal.pone.0059048. Epub 2013 Mar 12

[65] Newman SA, Miller NR. Optic tract syndrome. Neuro-ophthalmologic considerations. Archives of Ophthalmology. 1983;**101**:1241-1250

[66] Gammal TE, Brooks B, Harbour R, Kline L, Jacob P. MR of uncommon congenital and vascular lesions of the intracranial visual pathways. Neuroradiology. 1990;**32**:488-491

[67] Margo CE, Hamed LM, McCarty J. Congenital optic tract syndrome. Archives of Ophthalmology. 1991;**109**:1120-1122

[68] Hatsukawa Y, Fujio T, Nishikawa M, Taylor D. Congenital optic tract hypoplasia. Journal of AAPOS. 2015;**19**(4):383-385. DOI: 10.1016/j.jaapos.2015.03.018. Epub 2015 Jul 27

[69] Marsh-Tootle WL, Harb E, Hou W, Zhang Q, Anderson HA, Weise K, Norton TT, Gwiazda J, Hyman L. For the correction of myopia evaluation trial (COMET) study group. Optic nerve tilt, crescent, ovality, and torsion in a multi-ethnic cohort of young adults with and without myopia. Investigative Ophthalmology & Visual Science. 2017;**58**(7):3158-3171. DOI: 10.1167/iovs.16-20860

[70] American Academy of Ophthalmology. Basic and Clinical Science Course. Section 5: Neuroophthalmology. San Francisco, CA: American Academy of Ophthalmology; 2014. pp. 135-140

[71] Dutton JJ. Gliomas of the anterior visual pathway. Survey of Ophthalmology. 1994;**38**:427-452

[72] Rush JA, Younge BR, Campbell RJ, et al. Optic glioma: Long-term follow-up of 85 histologically verified cases. Ophthalmology. 1982;**89**:1213-1219

[73] Louis DN, Perry A, Reifenberger G, et al. The 2016 World Health Organization classification of tumors of the central nervous system: A summary. Acta Neuropathologica. 2016;**131**:803-820

[74] Ediriwickrema LS, Miller NR. Tumors of the optic nerve and its sheath. International Ophthalmology Clinics. 2018;**58**:237-260

[75] Miller NR. Optic gliomas: Past, present, and future. Journal of Neuro-Ophthalmology. 2016;**36**:460-473

[76] Miller NR. Primary tumours of the optic nerve and its sheath. Eye. 2004;**18**:1026-1037

[77] Brodsky MC. The Apparently Blind Infant In Pediatric Neuro-Ophthalmology. New York, NY: Springer; 2016. pp. 34-43

[78] Bandopadhaya P, Dagi L, Robinson N, et al. Morning glory disc anomaly in association with ipsilateral optic nerve glioma. Archives of Ophthalmology. 2012;**130**:1082

[79] Brodsky MC. The "pseudo-CSF" signal of orbital optic glioma on magnetic resonance imaging: A signature of neurofibromatosis. Survey of Ophthalmology. 1993;**38**:213-218

[80] Stern J, Jakobiec FA, Housepian EM. The architecture of optic nerve gliomas with and without neurofibromatosis. Archives of Ophthalmology. 1980;**98**:505-511

[81] Myron Y, Sassani JW. Chapter 13: Optic nerve. In: Ocular Pathology. 7th ed. London: W.B. Saunders; 2015. pp. 441e4-465e4. DOI: 10.1016/B978-1-4557-2874-9.00013-2

[82] Spicer GJ, Kazim M, Glass LR, et al. Accuracy of MRI in defining tumor-free margin in optic nerve glioma surgery. Ophthalmic Plastic and Reconstructive Surgery. 2013;**29**:277-280

[83] Yanoff M, Davis R, Zimmerman LE. Juvenile pilocytic astrocytoma ("glioma") of optic nerve: Clinicopathologic study of 63 cases. In: Jakobiec FA, editor. Ocular and Adnexal Tumors. Birmingham, AL: Aesculapius; 1978. p. 685

[84] Revere KE, Katowitz WR, Katowitz JA, et al. Childhood optic nerve glioma: Vision loss due to biopsy. Ophthalmic Plastic and Reconstructive Surgery. 2017;**33**:S107-S109

[85] Tow SL, Chandela S, Miller NR, et al. Long-term prognosis in children with gliomas of the anterior visual pathway. Pediatric Neurology. 2003;**28**:262-270

[86] Parsa CF, Hoyt WF, Lesser RL, et al. Spontaneous regression of optic gliomas. Thirteen cases documented by serial neuroimaging. Archives of Ophthalmology. 2001;**119**:516-529

[87] Parentin F, Rabusin M, Zannaro F, et al. Chemotherapy for optic nerve glioma in a child with neurofibromatosis type-1. Neuro-Ophthalmology. 2008;**32**:159-162

[88] Falsini B, Chiaretti A, Barone G, et al. Total nerve growth factor as a visual rescue strategy in pediatric optic gliomas: A pilot study including electrophysiology. Neurorehabilitation and Neural Repair. 2011;**25**:512-520

[89] McDonnell P, Miller NR. Chiasmatic and hypothalamic extension of optic nerve glioma. Archives of Ophthalmology. 1983;**101**:1412-1415

[90] Marwaha G, Macklis R, Singh AD. Radiation therapy: Orbital tumors. Developments in Ophthalmology. 2013;**52**:94-101

[91] Taveras JM, Mount LA, Wood EH. The value of radiation therapy in the management of glioma of the optic nerves and chiasm. Radiology. 1956;**66**:518-528

[92] Throuvalas N, Bataini P, Ennuyer A. Les gliomes du chiasma et du nerf optique: L'apport de la radiotherapie transcutanée dans leur traitement [Gliomas of the chiasm and optic

nerve: The role of external radiation therapy in their treatment]. Bulletin du Cancer Association Française Pour L'étude du Cancer. 1969;**56**:231-264

[93] Wolter JR. Large optic nerve glioma removed by the transconjunctival approach. Journal of Pediatric Ophthalmology. 1973;**10**:142-146

[94] Althekair FY. Debulking optic nerve gliomas for disfiguring proptosis: A globe-sparing approach by lateral orbitotomy alone. In: Presented as a Poster at the 42nd Annual Meeting of the North American Neuro-Ophthalmology Society; Tucson, AZ; February 28, 2016

[95] Spoor TC, Kennerdell JS, Martinez Z, et al. Malignant gliomas of the optic nerve pathways. American Journal of Ophthalmology. 1980;**89**:284-292

[96] Bailey P, Cushing H. A Classification of the Tumour of the Glioma 5: Group on a Histogenetic Basis with a Correlated Study of Prognosis. Philadelphia: Lippincott; 1926. pp. 26-48, 54-56

[97] Karch SB, Urich H. Medulloepithelioma: Definition of an entity. Journal of Neuropathology & Experimental Neurology. 1972;**31**:27-53

[98] Nakamura Y, Becker LE, Mancer K, Gillespie R. Peripheral medulloepithelioma. Acta Neuropathology (Berlin). 1982;**57**:137-142

[99] Chidambaram B, Santosh V, Balasubramanian V. Medulloepithelioma of the optic nerve with intradural extension: Report of two cases and a review of the literature. Child's Nervous System. 2000;**16**:329-333

[100] Chavez M, Mafee MF, Castillo B, et al. Medulloepithelioma of the optic nerve. Journal of Pediatric Ophthalmology and Strabismus. 2004;**41**:48-52

[101] McLendon RE, Kros JM, Bruner J, et al. Oligodendrogliomas. In: McLendon RE, Rosenblum MK, Bigner DD, editors. Russell and Rubinstein's Pathology of Tumors of the Nervous System. 7th ed. London: Hodder Arnold; 2006. pp. 167-186

[102] Hedges TR III. Tumors of neuroectodermal origin. In: Miller NR, Newman NJ, Biousse V, Kerrison JB, editors. Walsh and Hoyt's Clinical Neuro-Ophthalmology. 6th ed. Philadelphia, PA: Lippincott Williams & Wilkins; 2005. pp. 1439-1442

[103] Lucarini C, Tomei G, Gaini SM, et al. A case of optic nerve oligodendroglioma associated with an orbital non-Hodgkin's lymphoma in adult. Case report. Journal of Neurosurgery Science. 1990;**34**:319-321

[104] Offret H, Gregoire-Cassoux N, Frau E, et al. Solitary oligodendroglioma of the optic nerve. Apropos of a case. Journal Français d'Ophtalmologie. 1995;**18**:158-163

[105] Rolston JD, Han SJ, Cotter JA, et al. Gangliogliomas of the optic pathway. Journal of Clinical Neuroscience. 2014;**21**:2244-2249

[106] Gritzman MCD, Snyckers FD, Proctor NS. Ganglioglioma of the optic nerve. A case report. South African Medical Journal. 1983;**63**:863-865

[107] Bergin DJ, Johnson TE, Spencer WH, et al. Ganglioglioma of the optic nerve. American Journal of Ophthalmology. 1988;**105**:146-149

[108] Kerr DJ, Scheithauer BW, Miller GM, et al. Hemangioblastoma of the optic nerve: Case report. Neurosurgery. 1995;**36**:573-581

[109] Simpson RK Jr, Harper RL, Kirkpatrick JB, Cooper B. Schwannoma of the optic sheath. Journal of Neuro-Ophthalmology. 1987;**7**:219-222

[110] Kim DS, Choi JU, Yang KH, Jung JM. Optic sheath schwannomas: Report of two cases. Child's Nervous System. 2002;**18**:684-689

[111] Kinoshita Y, Kurosaki M, Kamitani H, Watanabe T. Schwannoma originating in the optic canal. Acta Neurochirurgica. 2008;**150**:89-90

[112] Birkholz ES, Lee AG, Nerad JA, Lane KA, Bilyk JR. A pregnant pause. Survey of Ophthalmology. 2010;**55**:162-168

[113] Russel DS, Rubenstein EJ. Pathology of Tumours of the Nervous System. 4th ed. London: Edward Arnold; 1977. pp. 372-379

[114] Haga Y, Shoji H, Oguro K, Mori S, Kawai T, Shinoda S, et al. Intra-cerebral schwannoma—Case report. Neurologia Medico-Chirurgica (Tokyo). 1997;**37**:551-555

[115] Rootman J, Goldberg C, Robertson W. Primary orbital schwannomas. The British Journal of Ophthalmology. 1982;**66**:194-204

[116] Civit T, Freppel S. Intraorbital Schwannomas and solitary neurofibromas. Neuro-Chirurgie. 2010;**56**:137-141

[117] Dutton JJ. Optic nerve sheath meningiomas. Survey of Ophthalmology. 1992;**37**:167-183

[118] Miller NR. New concepts in the diagnosis and management of optic nerve sheath meningioma. Journal of Neuro-Ophthalmology. 2006;**26**:200-208

[119] Shapey J, Sabin HI, Danesh-Meyer HV, et al. Diagnosis and management of optic nerve sheath meningiomas. Journal of Clinical Neuroscience. 2013;**20**:1045-1056

[120] Bosch MM, Wichmann WW, Boltshauser E, et al. Optic nerve sheath meningiomas in patients with neurofibromatosis type 2. Archives of Ophthalmology. 2006;**124**:379-385

[121] Schick U, Dott U, Hassler W. Surgical management of meningiomas involving the optic nerve sheath. Journal of Neurosurgery. 2004;**101**:951-959

[122] Christmas NJ, Mead MD, Richardson EP, Albert DM. Secondary optic nerve tumors. Survey of Ophthalmology. 1991;**36**(3):196-206

Chapter 4

Optic Nerve Changes in Diabetic Retinopathy

Andi Arus Victor

Additional information is available at the end of the chapter

http://dx.doi.org/10.5772/intechopen.81221

Abstract

Diabetic retinopathy (DR) is a devastating sight-threatening complication of diabetes mellitus (DM). Besides damaging the vascular system of the retina, DM will also destruct the tissue surrounding the retina, including the optic nerve. DR impairs the optic nerve by damaging its conduction and integrity. There are few clinical manifestations of optic nerve changes in DR such as diabetic papillopathy, neovascularization of optic disc, and optic nerve atrophy. These involve metabolic alterations related to DM, production of advanced glycation end products (AGEs), oxidative stress, and hemodynamic changes. Diagnostic tests including visual evoked potential (VEP) and optical coherence tomography (OCT) can detect functional and structural changes. This finding is important as it may reflect the early loss of retinal ganglion cell axons. As the neuronal loss is irreversible, it is pivotal to be able to screen these nervous system changes in the early stage of DR and prevent further deterioration.

Keywords: diabetes mellitus, diabetic papillopathy, diabetic retinopathy, neovascularization of optic disc, optical coherence tomography, optic nerve, optic atrophy, visual evoked potential

1. Introduction

Diabetic retinopathy (DR), a devastating sight-threatening complication of diabetes mellitus (DM), is one of the most prevalent health diseases worldwide with an incidence of 6.9% [1–3]. The number of people with diabetes is estimated to rise from 171 million in 2000 to 366 million in 2030. A study by Jin et al. in DM type 2 population showed that within 5 years, the cumulative incidence of DR was 46.9% with 13.9% population suffering from severe nonproliferative DR (NPDR) and 4.6% from proliferative DR (PDR). Hence, more people will be at risk of developing DR and in danger of losing their sight [4, 5].

DM endangers sight by damaging the neurovascular system of the eye, including the optic nerve [6, 7]. The damages include changes in angioarchitecture, blood flow and degenerative loss of neural tissue, morphological changes, changed protein expression, and changed neurotransmission and neurotransmitters [6–9]. Recently, not so many studies have been conducted to elucidate damage due to DM and DR in the optic nerve and central visual pathway. We hypothesize that optic nerve damage occurs due to few processes in DM. Such processes are metabolic alteration, oxidative stress, and ischemia [10]. These changes could be detected via modalities such as visual evoked potential, biomicroscopy, and fundus photography [11–13]. These changes usually occur after persistent metabolic alterations, which may lead to late detection [2, 14]. Therefore, early detection of optic nerve involvement in DR may be beneficial to provide timely recognition and management for patients at greater risk of DR progression [14].

2. Pathophysiology

There are few processes in DR affecting the optic nerve. Such processes are metabolic alterations related to DM, production of advanced glycation end products (AGEs), oxidative stress, and hemodynamic changes. These processes will be discussed in detail below.

2.1. Metabolic alterations

Findings from animal studies suggest that neurodegeneration in DR is caused by both diminished insulin receptor signaling and systemic hyperglycemia [15–17]. Insulin plays an important role, as insulin receptors in the retina stimulate neuronal development, growth, and anabolic synthesis [18, 19]. Therefore, a defect in insulin function either due to a low level of insulin or impaired sensitivity would hamper neuroretinal cells' survival. As diabetes progresses, retinal neurons start to degenerate by apoptosis within weeks after the onset [20, 21]. Metabolic alteration and hormonal factors might affect balance of some mediators including growth factors, cytokines, inflammatory, and adhesion molecules [22]. These alterations result in abnormal capillary permeability, apoptosis of capillary cells, and angiogenesis [23].

Metabolic alteration also damages neural conduction in the postretinal central visual pathway [10]. A recent study in diabetic rats showed that there is reduction of Na^+/K^+/ATPase enzyme in the optic nerve [24]. This enzyme is important for maintaining sodium potassium gradient within cells and controls the membrane axon depolarization/repolarization. When impaired, it suggests that the neuronal conduction and integrity are damaged.

2.2. Advanced glycation end products

Hyperglycemia induces reaction of sugar and protein via Maillard reaction and produces advanced glycation end products (AGEs) [25, 26]. AGEs play a huge role in complications of DM as it triggers further oxidative stress and vascular cross-linking and activates pro-inflammatory cytokines [20, 21]. Neriyanuri et al. reported that AGEs were independent predictors of development of DR in addition to blood glucose and glycated hemoglobin [14].

AGEs are long-lasting, irreversible products that can modify blood vessel elasticity [25]. High-level AGEs in the optic disc affect elasticity of lamina cribrosa. As the intraocular pressure increases, cribriform plates become unable to bear the strain. This condition may develop into glaucoma in DR [27].

2.3. Oxidative stress

Hyperglycemia stimulates increased flux through the glycolytic and tricarboxylic acid cycle pathways, hence resulting in excessive electrons within mitochondria [28]. These electrons would react with oxygen and form reactive oxygen species (ROS). Since mitochondria as cells' powerhouse also generate ROS on their own, they are also the first ones to be damaged by increased ROS. This results in reduced mitochondrial energy production, later causing loss of cellular and tissue function [29].

Oxidative stress also contributes to neural retinal ganglion cell and optic nerve injury through the impairment of L-glutamate/L-aspartate transporter (GLAST), which increases extracellular accumulation of glutamate and promotes excitotoxicity [30–32]. Glutamate is a neurotransmitter that plays a role in the regulation of neurohormonal activity and is found in high levels in the central nervous system. Upon stimulation of nerve cells, glutamate molecules are released from the glutamatergic synaptic vesicles and cause depolarization of the postsynaptic neuronal membrane, which generates signal. Accumulated glutamate in the synaptic space is then collected by adjacent astrocytes, afterward being broken down into glutamine [21].

In patients with DR, glutamate accumulates in extracellular space due to the following mechanisms: (1) reduction of Müller cell–specific enzyme glutamine synthetase, which converts glutamate to glutamine; (2) decrease in the retinal ability to oxidize glutamate to α-ketoglutarate; and (3) impairment of glutamate uptake by the glial cells [29]. The accumulation of glutamate results in overactivity of ionotropic glutamate receptors, such as α-amino-3-hydroxyl-5-methyl-4-isoxazole-propionate (AMPA) and N-methyl-D-aspartate (NMDA) receptors, which later causes uncontrolled intracellular calcium response in postsynaptic neurons and eventually cell death [33, 34]. Recent studies suggest that glutamate excitotoxicity results in apoptotic degenerative lesions [25]. Glutamate toxicity also causes depletion of glutathione, which is an antioxidant, thus contributing to oxidative stress [35].

A recent study in diabetic rats also showed marked increase in oxidative stress level shown by malondialdehyde (MDA) level in the optic nerve and visual cortex. In addition, they also found reduced antioxidant, glutathione (GSH), in both the optic nerve and visual cortex [24]. These results suggest significant oxidative stress in the optic nerve and visual cortex along with impairment in neuronal conduction and integrity. Other studies have also found similar result, showing impaired retrograde and anterograde axonal transport in the optic nerve of diabetic rats along with retinal ganglion cell axonopathy [36, 37]. A study by Sokol et al. showed that when induced with ischemia, myelinated axons degenerated and became disordered [38]. Further changes are swollen and collapsed axons, and by 90th minute, myelin sheaths were fragmented. Joachim et al. found axonal damage and gliosis of the optic nerve after ocular ischemia. Renner et al. found damaged optic nerve in an ischemic rat model. Histologic examination revealed demyelination and subsequent loss of myelin sheaths after ischemia [39]. In addition, they also found marked microglia activation, upregulation of astrocytes, reduction of myelin basic protein and myelin oligodendrocyte glycoprotein (MOG), as well as the reduction in oligodendrocytes [40]. The optic nerve structure was also affected as neurofilament was found to be distorted after 21 days of ischemia/reperfusion induction. Ischemia also seemed to impair neuronal immune system as the study found destroyed astroglia structure, hence leaving the nerve tissue susceptible to insults, i.e., oxidative stress [40].

2.4. Hemodynamic changes

Chronic hyperglycemia damages the retinal blood vessels and causes pericyte loss due to elevated sorbitol level. These result in involution of the vascular changes in microcirculation and loss of normal capillary exchange [12–14]. Microvascular anomalies and chronic inflammation may develop dysfunctional barriers permitting leakage of inflammatory molecules and immune cells from systemic circulation and cause further deterioration of the tissue [12, 41].

Another process that plays a major part in DR is capillary degeneration due to weakness and dilation of capillary walls' saccular outpouching, commonly known as microaneurysms. Rupture of these microaneurysms leads to leakage of endovascular products, including blood [9]. In DR, blood viscosity was significantly higher, thus resulting in reductions in blood flow. Persistent uncorrected blood flow causes chronic mild hypoperfusion, which might lead to ischemia and a rise in waste products [42, 43].

Accumulation of these molecules and cells leads to retinal occlusion, which later progresses into hypoxia [44]. Hypoxia results in upregulation of vascular endothelial growth factor (VEGF) platelet adhesiveness, erythrocyte aggregation, serum lipids, and fibrinolysis [45, 46]. VEGF promotes new blood vessel growth resulting in abnormal neovascularization [47].

3. Clinical manifestation

There are few clinical manifestations of optic nerve damage related to DM and DR that can be observed. Those are diabetic papillopathy, neovascularization of optic disc, and optic nerve atrophy [48]. Those will be discussed further below.

3.1. Diabetic papillopathy

3.1.1. Definition

Diabetic papillopathy (DP) is an ocular manifestation of both type 1 and type 2 DM characterized by unilateral or bilateral hyperemic disc swelling with minimal or no optic nerve dysfunction, which generally resolves without medical intervention [49, 50]. Patients with DP are often asymptomatic, but may sometimes experience transient decrease in visual acuity [50]. It is usually self-limiting and tends to resolve over a period of 2–10 months with the average time of 3.7 months, leaving minimal sequelae [51, 52]. Visual acuity generally recovers to better than 20/30 in most patients [53].

DP typically affects young people with type 1 DM, but it has also been reported to occur in elderly patients with type 2 DM. The prevalence of DP in both types of DM is 0.5% and the percentage of DP patients presenting with nonproliferative diabetic retinopathy (NPDR) is higher than in the proliferative diabetic retinopathy (PDR) [49].

3.1.2. *Pathophysiology*

The pathophysiology of diabetic papillopathy remains poorly understood and several theories have been suggested [49]. Some researchers suggest that DP is a subtype of anterior ischemic optic neuropathy (AION), but there are different features between DP and AION that others argue that it is a completely different pathological process [49, 50]. For instance, DP is an asymptomatic optic disc edema, whereas AION is an acute optic disc infarction [54, 55]. Researchers support the argument that the pathophysiology of DP is distinguishable from AION [50]. A study evaluating fluroangiographic aspects by Brancato et al. showed robust leakage of fluorescein, suggesting that DP is a local nonhypotensive vasculopathy [56]. These findings are supported by Bayraktar et al. and Regillo et al., who showed notable telangiectatic vasculature and fluroangiographic hyperfluorescence [54, 57]. Meanwhile, case studies of AION by Hayreh et al. and Shin et al. demonstrated notable filling defects in fluroangiography [55, 58]. These findings of AION contrast with the hyperfluorescence that has been noted in cases of DP.

In patients with DP, the degree of DR tends to be mild. Regillo et al. observed that DP might be a separate entity rather than extension of DR [57]. Otherwise, a case series by Ostri et al. reported that three out of four patients with DP who already had DR before proceeded to develop high-risk PDR. This condition is called "early worsening phenomenon of DR " where progression of retinopathy and papillopathy was accelerated, while adaptation was remarkably slow in the very first year [59]. Bayraktar et al. also reported two cases of nonproliferative diabetic retinopathy (NPDR), which later on were also diagnosed as having DP. A 3-month follow-up showed that retinopathy worsened and developed into proliferative diabetic retinopathy (PDR) [54]. Lubow et al. found that two of three patients with DP subsequently developed PDR and vitreous hemorrhage [60]. Hayreh et al. reported similar findings and observed three patients with DP, who later on were also diagnosed as having PDR [55]. Hence, DP should be considered as a risk factor for progression to PDR and patients should be observed closely taking into account this possibility [54].

Early DP study by Appen et al. hypothesized that DP patients sustain a local vasculopathy of the optic disc, presumably in relation to diabetes [61]. This vasculopathy induces transient leakage of fluid, which results in disc edema. The authors also suggest that the presence of edema causes axoplasmic flow turmoil. An earlier study by Freund et al. showed that prolonged hyperglycemia and anoxia due to the failure of glucose utilization cause damages to the optic nerve [62]. Recent study by Slagle et al. suggested that clinically visible interstitial edema of the optic nerve head due to vascular hyperpermeability initiates the pathology of DP [50].

Slagle et al. elucidate that tissue perfusion depends on two main factors: (1) the ability of the blood to reach the tissue through patent vessels and (2) the dispersion of nutrients to the tissue via fluid movement through the capillary bed. There are four primary forces that determine perfusion: (1) capillary pressure, (2) interstitial fluid pressure, (3) plasma colloid osmotic pressure, and (4) interstitial fluid colloid osmotic pressure [50]. The authors hypothesized that impairment in the transportation and reabsorption of fluid through the capillary walls causes capillary vasostatic perfusion pathology. Diabetes causes damages to vascular endothelium, which leads to initial vasculopathy characterized by increased vascular permeability [53]. Along with loss of pericytes, this causes hemodynamics and autoregulation derangements [53, 63].

In the early stage of diabetic vasculopathy, the hyperpermeability of diabetic capillaries causes excessive protein to spill from the plasma into the interstitium. This leads to the offsets of physiological osmotic gradient, creating deficiency in fluid reabsorption on the venule end of the capillary bed. Edema occurs when the lymphatic system is unable to correct this imbalance [50]. The typical transient initial edematous course of DP suggests that optic nerve capillaries are susceptible to this vasculopathy. Edema compresses vessels leading to ischemia as well as stagnates and prolongs cellular exposure to toxic effects from free radicals and cellular waste. In addition, edema might also compress nerve fibers causing axoplasmic flow derangements [61, 62, 64]. These hypotheses would explain the reported fluroangiographic hyperfluorescence in DP, its relatively benign nature compared to AION, and its transient course [50].

In the later stage of DP, ischemia may result from leukostasis-derived capillary occlusion due to retinal leukostasis effect and thickened capillary basement membranes, which affect retinal capillary endothelial function, perfusion, angiogenesis, and vascular permeability [64]. This results in a clinical picture resembling more like traditional AION sequelae with optic atrophy [50].

3.1.3. Clinical features

The main features of DP are painless visual loss, macular edema, disc hyperfluorescence on fluroangiography, and significant visual improvement after treatment [49, 54]. Differential diagnoses include infection, inflammation, metastatic infiltration, hypertension, and papilledema [52, 57, 65].

3.1.4. Diagnostic studies

Certain diagnostic criteria have to be met in order to recognize diabetic papillopathy. The current accepted diagnostic criteria include (1) confirmed diagnosis of diabetes; (2) unilateral or bilateral presence of optic disc edema; (3) normal intracranial pressure; (4) absence of inflammation, infiltration, or infection in the optic disc; and (5) a lack of substantial optic nerve dysfunction [50, 51]. Supportive examination to confirm DP includes fluorescein angiography (FA), orbital magnetic resonance imaging (MRI), and blood tests ranging from serum angiotensin-converting enzyme (ACE), antinuclear antibody (ANA), vitamin B12, folate, erythrocyte sedimentation rate (ESR), C reactive protein (CRP) to fluorescent treponemal antibody test [49].

3.1.5. Treatment

There is no evidence that the resolution of DP and the prevention of permanent visual loss can be promoted by definitive treatment. As stated before, in most cases, the edema resolves within a few months (average of 3.7 months) to no visual impairment [49]. Because of its self-limiting nature, the most common management is serial examinations. However, due to potential visual sequelae noted in certain cases, more efforts have to be made to identify at-risk patients and effective treatment to prevent this sequela.

Although originally thought to be related to glycemic control, systemic glucose manipulation has not shown any benefits in DP [51]. Hence, how diabetes treatment should be titrated to protect visual function in DP remains uncertain [59]. Current treatment aims to reduce disc edema in DP, including intravitreal anti-VEGF, which has been shown to increase visual acuity and decrease disc edema, and also periocular corticosteroids, which stabilizes the blood-ocular barrier at the disc [65–69].

3.2. Neovascularization of optic disc

3.2.1. Definition

Diabetic retinopathy is often associated with neovascular proliferation due to ischemia in the retina and release of angiogenic factors. These conditions cause neovascularization of the optic disc (NVD), also neovascularization elsewhere (NVE) [70, 71]. Patients with NVD have a poor visual prognosis due to high incidence of complication, such as vitreous hemorrhage, fibrous proliferation, and traction retinal detachment. NVD occurring in DR can be accompanied by NVE and NVI (neovascularization of the iris), which later on may develop into neovascular glaucoma (NVG), which is an optic neuropathy defined by changes in the optic nerve and associated with visual field defects and elevated intraocular pressure [70]. Recent studies have shown that PDR is the leading cause of neovascular glaucoma [72].

3.2.2. Pathophysiology

In DR, capillary occlusion and reduced perfusion in retina provoke cascade events related to hypoxia and lead to angiogenesis. Normally, pro-angiogenic factors (VEGF and angiopoietin-2) and antiangiogenic factors (pigment epithelium-derived growth factor) are in equilibrium [71]. Imbalance between those factors might trigger activation, proliferation, and migration of endothelial cells and pericytes and lead to neovascularization [71–73]. VEGF is produced in a variety of neuroretinal cells and plays a major part in promoting intraocular neovascularization. Inflammatory cytokines interleukin-6 (IL-6) is also correlated with the degree of neovascularization patients. Other potential pro-angiogenic factors include basic fibroblast growth factor (bFGF), transforming growth factor-beta 1 and -beta 2, nitric oxide, and endothelin-1 [73].

The new vessels at the disc can bleed spontaneously or with minimal trauma. The blood spills into the retina and between the retina and vitreous causing vitreoretinal hemorrhage. This condition attracts fibroglial elements and finally resulting in separation between inner layers of the retina and the underlying retinal pigment epithelium, which is known as tractional retinal detachment [3]. NVD and NVI do not always develop into NVG, although neovascularization always develops prior to intraocular pressure increase. This is primarily due to fibrovascular membrane that develops on the iris and iridocorneal angle, which later causes anterior synechiae, angle closure, and intraocular pressure elevation [49, 74].

3.2.3. Clinical features

In early stages of neovascularization, patients may be asymptomatic or may present with low vision. Ocular findings can be subtle in early stage, so case history and complete ocular examination are important to make early diagnosis [71–73].

3.2.4. Diagnostic studies

Fundus examination might trace the new vessels of the optic disc and reveal glaucomatous optic nerve damage [73–75]. In fluorescein angiography (FA), leakage from damaged vessels could be detected before development of visible neovascularization. Even though FA can aid early detection, the test is not always available [73, 76]. Using OCT angiography (OCTA), neovascularization around the optic disc at the level of the vitreous cavity might be observed in a faster and safer way [75]. Electroretinography and retinal angiography can be necessary to determine the origin of neovascularization in the retina. Meanwhile, gonioscopy is a low-cost and fast test, which can reveal NVI [73, 76].

3.2.5. Treatment

Early diagnosis will enable early treatment and prevent blindness due to optic nerve neovascularization. Tight glycemic control is also important [75]. Medical intervention to prevent further visual loss related to NVG is associated with lowering the IOP levels using topical β-adrenergic antagonists, α-2 agonists, and carbonic anhydrase inhibitors. Topical corticosteroid can also be used to reduce inflammation [73]. The main treatment for preventing NVD and NVE in DR is laser photocoagulation. Panretinal photocoagulation laser therapy in early stages is beneficial by inhibiting and reversing neovascularization [74]. Use of anti-VEGF, cyclophotocoagulation, cryotherapy, and surgery are among other therapeutic options.

3.3. Optic nerve atrophy

3.3.1. Definition

Optic nerve atrophy is the end result of any disease that causes optic nerve damage anywhere along the path from the retina to the lateral geniculate. Degeneration of axon will manifest as changes in color and structure of the optic disc. It is associated with variable degrees of visual dysfunction, including congenital, vascular, metabolic, inflammatory condition, trauma, and neoplasm [77, 78].

3.3.2. Pathophysiology

Optic nerve atrophy could result from many processes related to DM and DR. Such processes include neurodegeneration, oxidative stress, and ischemia. It may also develop as a result of optic nerve abnormalities mentioned above. Further study should be carried out to distinguish whether optic nerve atrophy occurs as a result of DR or complications of laser photocoagulation [10, 24, 36].

3.3.3. Clinical features

The main symptom of optic atrophy is vision loss. In optic nerve atrophy, axon loss and myelin shrinkage will show the pallor-appearing disc, widening of the optic cup, and decreased Kestenbaum index (less than 6) [78].

3.3.4. Diagnostic studies

Optic nerve atrophy is easy to diagnose, but finding the etiology is challenging. Further diagnostic test is necessary to identify the etiology of optic atrophy. Imaging study, such as ultrasonography, CT, and MRI, is used depending on the disease process. Other diagnostic tests are visual acuity testing, color vision testing, contrast sensitivity test, visual field testing, electroretinography, optical coherence tomography, and visual evoked response [78].

3.3.5. Treatment

No proven treatment is able to return the function of atrophic optic nerve. Experts believe that treatment initiated before the development of optic nerve atrophy can be very useful to save the remaining function. The goal of primary intervention is to prevent axon degeneration by finding and treating the cause of optic atrophy. In diabetic patients, tight glycemic control and early detection of DR are very important. If the main problem is found and well-treated, further damage can be prevented [78].

4. Diagnostic approach for detecting optic nerve changes in diabetic retinopathy

Various examination methods have been used to detect functional and structural optic nerve changes in patients with diabetic retinopathy.

4.1. Visual functional test

4.1.1. Visual acuity

As has been known, neurodegeneration is a progressive loss of structure and function of neurons. The quality of visual acuity (VA) depends on the normal condition of visual pathway. Visual acuity test is the standard test of visual function. There are two commonly used tools for evaluating VA, including the Snellen VA chart and the Early Treatment Diabetic Retinopathy Study (ETDRS) VA chart. The Snellen VA chart is a frequently used chart for measuring VA. This consists of different type, size, and number of letters in each row. In contrast, ETDRS-VA chart has an equal number of characters per row with relatively uniform legibility. Some studies agree that ETDRS-VA chart has more advantages over the Snellen VA chart. Moreover, besides VA tests, some experts suggested that psychophysical tests, such as visual field and contrast sensitivity test, should also be evaluated in DR patients with optic nerve complication. They found that those examinations were more sensitive than VA test only [13].

4.1.2. Contrast sensitivity

Contrast sensitivity is a test of the inner retina, with different spatial frequencies in specific neural pathways [13]. There is no algorithm to define the pattern of contrast sensitivity alteration in the early stage of DR. Adachi, Jochim, and Renner. observed reduced contrast sensitivity only at single low spatial frequency in cases of non–insulin-dependent diabetes mellitus without DR [79–81]. Meanwhile, Joltikov et al. and Safi et al reported decline in contrast sensitivity at all spatial frequencies early in the course of diabetic retinal sensory neuropathy [14, 82]. Joltikov et al. suggested that contrast sensitivity might be the most sensitive test for detection of subtle functional impairment in diabetic patients with or without retinopathy. In addition, contrast sensitivity test is more practical than electroretinography [13]. However, longitudinal study showed that reduced contrast sensitivity in the earlier stage of the disease might be reversible [82].

4.1.3. Visual fields

Another visual function affected by neurodegeneration is visual fields. A common test for evaluating the visual field in diabetic retinopathy is perimetry. Various perimetry methods have been applied including white-on-white standard automated perimetry (SAP), frequency doubling technology perimetry (FDP), short-wavelength automated perimetry (SWAP), and rarebit perimetry (RBP) [83, 84]. Bengtsson et al. suggested that SAP and SWAP are more sensitive to neuroretinal impairment than ETDRS-VA chart [85]. Safi et al. reported that by using microperimetry, it might detect a reduction of foveal sensitivity in diabetic patients with preclinical stage of DR [82].

4.1.4. Color vision test

Many color vision tests have been assessed in diabetic patients with and without retinopathy diabetes, including Lanthony desaturated D-15, Farnsworth-Munsell 100-Hue, and chromatography tests. However, studies recommended that Farnsworth-Munsell 100-hue test has higher sensitivity than the other tests. This test has been recommended as a screening test for DR patients [82].

4.1.5. Visual evoked potential

Visual evoked potential (VEP) is a noninvasive test that evaluates the visual pathways by recording the electric signal in response to a bright flash of light [86, 87]. Changes of amplitudes and latencies in VEP reflects impairment in ganglion cells and optic nerve [88]. Clinical conditions that cause a delay in VEP latencies include papillitis, neuritis, toxic optic neuropathies, multiple sclerosis, glaucoma, and conditions affecting conducting media [89].

Khatoon observed that the pattern of VEP responses may provide early diagnosis of optic nerve involvement in DR and define the prognosis [88]. Onset of diabetes blood glucose control might affect the result of VEP [89]. In diabetic patients, VEP amplitude was reduced progressively with an increase of latency as the years pass [87]. Farisa et al. showed that P100 latency was prolonged among diabetic patients compared to nondiabetic subjects [88].

Progressive delay in VEP latency reflects damage of ganglion cell, even before the first ophthalmoscopically noticeable signs arise. VEP should be done as a screening tool for detecting optic nerve involvement in DR. Thus, early and proper management can be done to prevent further ocular damage [88].

4.2. Structural test

4.2.1. Fundus photography

Fundus photography is a noninvasive examination for documenting clinical signs and monitoring the progression or improvement of retinal diseases over time. One of the purposes of fundus photography is screening DR in diabetic patients. This method is useful for illustrating normal and abnormal morphology of the retina [90, 91]. Some signs of neurodegeneration in DR patients could be screened by fundus photography, including papilledema and macular edema. However, the result of fundus photography is a two-dimensional image; thus, it is difficult to accurately assess the detailed morphology of the retina leading to a high false-positive rate. In addition, in the condition of vitreous hemorrhage or low-quality image, some part of the retina could not be evaluated [10, 48].

4.2.2. Fundus fluorescein angiography

Fundus fluorescein angiography (FFA) is an invaluable imaging method demonstrating an interaction of fluorescent within the anatomic structure of ocular fundus. FFA is the gold standard in evaluating retinal vascularization. FFA has early and late phase. Early phase demonstrates following the injection until complete filling of retinal arteries, arterioles, and capillaries, while the late phase demonstrates filling of veins until gradual elimination of the fluorescent from the retinal vasculature. Hypofluorescence occurs due to a vascular filling defect or a secondary condition of a blocking effect, while hyperfluorescence may occur due to fluorescein leakage, staining, or pooling [10, 24, 36].

4.2.3. Optical coherence tomography

Optical coherence tomography (OCT) is a high-resolution imaging modality to measure retinal morphology, including vitreoretinal interface, neurosensory retina, and subretinal space [48]. We can measure the retinal layer thickness and segmentation [92, 93]. OCT provides an accurate assessment with low specificity value [48]. OCT is divided into two types: spectral domain (SD) and time domain (TD) [2]. TD-OCT is mostly used in neuro-ophthalmology to measure peripapillary retinal nerve fiber layer (RNFL) thickness. Peripapillary RNFL thickness increases in disc edema and decreases in optic nerve atrophy [94]. The results of OCT can be used as a guide for making therapeutic decision.

4.2.4. Optical coherence tomography angiography

Optical coherence tomography angiography (OCT-A) is a three-dimensional noninvasive chorioretinal vascular imaging to observe the microvascular structures of new vessels, including

NVD and NVE [95]. OCT-A can analyze blood flow in the vessels without dye injections. In FFA, it sometimes showed artifacts due to dye leakage effect. OCT-A is superior to FFA in determining the number, course, size, and extension of NVD [96].

5. Conclusion

Changes in the optic nervous system may start prior to classic clinical manifestation of DR. The development of an integrated multimodal approach for detecting optic nerve involvement in DR is important for early diagnosis in preclinical stage DR and reducing diabetic complications.

Conflict of interest

There are no conflicts of interest in this chapter.

Author details

Andi Arus Victor

Address all correspondence to: arvimadao@yahoo.com

Department of Ophthalmology, Faculty of Medicine, Universitas Indonesia,
Cipto Mangunkusumo National General Hospital, Jakarta, Indonesia

References

[1] Abcouwer SF, Gardner TW. Diabetic retinopathy: Loss of neuroretinal adaptation to the diabetic metabolic environment. Annals of the New York Academy of Sciences. 2014;**1311**: 174-190. DOI: 10.1111/nyas.12412

[2] Mazumder AG, Chatterjee S, Chatterjee S, Gonzalez JJ, Bag S, Ghosh S, et al. Spectro-pathology-corroborated multimodal quantitative imaging biomarkers for neuroretinal degeneration in diabetic retinopathy. Journal of Clinical Ophthalmology. 2017;**11**:2073-2089. DOI: 10.2147/OPTH.S140110

[3] Nentwich MM, Ulbig MW. Diabetic retinopathy—ocular complications of diabetes mellitus. World Journal of Diabetes. 2015;**6**(3):489-499. DOI: 10.4239/wjd.v6.i3.489

[4] Wild S, Roglic G, Green A, Sicree R, King H. Global prevalence of diabetes. Diabetes Care. 2004;**27**(5):1047-1053. DOI: 10.2337/diacare.27.5.1047

[5] Wu L, Fernandez-Loaiza P, Sauma J, Hernandez-Bogantes E, Masis M. Classification of diabetic retinopathy and diabetic macular edema. World Journal of Diabetes. 2013;**4**(6):290-294. DOI: 10.4239/wjd.v4.i6.290

[6] Barber AJ, Lieth E, Khin SA, Antonetti DA, Buchanan AG, Gardner TW. Neural apoptosis in the retina during experimental and human diabetes. The Journal of Clinical Investigation. 1998;**102**(4):783-791

[7] Barber AJ, Gardner TW, Abcouwer SF. The significance of vascular and neural apoptosis to the pathology of diabetic retinopathy. Investigative Ophthalmology & Visual Science. 2011;**52**:1156-1163

[8] Chen X, Nie C, Gong Y, Zhang Y, Jin X, Wei S, et al. Peripapillary retinal nerve fiber layer changes in preclinical diabetic retinopathy: A meta-analysis. PLoS One. 2015;**10**(5):e0125919. DOI: 10.1371/journal.pone.0125919

[9] Pekel E, Tufaner G, Kaya H, Kasikci A, Deda G, Pekel G. Assessment of optic disc and ganglion cell layer in diabetes mellitus type 2. Medicine. 2017;**96**(29):e7556. DOI: 10.1097/MD.0000000000007556

[10] Gregori B, Galié E, Pro S, Clementi A, Accornero N. Luminance and chromatic visual evoked potentials in type I and II diabetes: Relationships with peripheral neuropathy. Neurological Sciences. 2006;**27**:323-327

[11] Zheng Y, He M, Congdon N. The worldwide epidemic of diabetic retinopathy. Indian Journal of Ophthalmology. 2012;**60**(5):428-431. DOI: 10.4103/0301-4738.100542

[12] Pemp B, Palkovits S, Howorka K, Pumprla J, Sacu S, Garhöfer G, et al. Correlation of retinal neurodegeneration with measures of peripheral autonomic neuropathy in type 1 diabetes. Acta Ophthalmologica. 2018:1-7. DOI: 10.1111/aos.13733. DOI: 10.1111/aos.13733

[13] Joltikov KA, deCastro VM, Davila JR, Anand R, Khan SM, Farbman N, et al. Multidimensional functional and structural evaluation reveals neuroretinal impairment in early diabetic retinopathy. Investigative Ophthalmology & Visual Science. 2017;**58**:BIO277-BIO290. DOI: 10.1167/iovs.17-21863

[14] Neriyanuri S, Pardhan S, Gella L, Pal SS, Ganesan S, Sharma T, et al. Retinal sensitivity changes associated with diabetic neuropathy in the absence of diabetic retinopathy. The British Journal of Ophthalmology. 2017;**101**(9):1174-1178. DOI: 10.1136/bjophthalmol-2016-309641

[15] Adams AJ, Bearse MA. Retinal neuropathy precedes vasculopathy in diabetes: A function-based opportunity for early treatment intervention? Clinical and Experimental Optometry. 2012;**95**(3):256-265

[16] Heng LZ, Comyn O, Peto T, Tadros C, Ng E, Sivaprasad S, et al. Diabetic retinopathy: Pathogenesis, clinical grading, management and future developments. Diabetic Medicine. 2013;**30**:640-650. DOI: 10.1111/dme.12089

[17] Jiao C, Abramoff MD, Lee K. Diabetes induced neurodegeneration in the retina and the brain of mice are associated and independent of microvasculopathy. Investigative Ophthalmology and Visual Science. 2017;**58**:5195

[18] Rajala RVS, Anderson RE. Rhodopsin-regulated insulin receptor signaling pathway in rod photoreceptor neurons. Molecular Neurobiology. 2010;**42**(1):39-47. DOI: 10.1007/s12035-010-8130-8

[19] Rajala RVS. Phosphoinositide 3-kinase signaling in the vertebrate retina. Journal of Lipid Research. 2010;**51**(1):4-22. DOI: 10.1194/jlr.R000232

[20] Stem MS, Gardner TW. Neurodegeneration in the pathogenesis of diabetic retinopathy: Molecular mechanisms and therapeutic implications. Current Medicinal Chemistry. 2014; **20**(26):3241-3250

[21] Kergoat H, Hérard ME, Lemay M. RGC sensitivity to mild systemic hypoxia. Investigative Ophthalmology & Visual Science. 2006;**47**(12):5423-5427. DOI: 10.1167/iovs.06-0602

[22] Abcouwer SF. Angiogenic factors and cytokines in diabetic retinopathy. Journal of Clinical and Cellular Immunology. 2013;**11**:1. DOI: 10.4172/2155-9899

[23] Victor AA, Sitompul R. Proliferative diabetic retinopathy: An overview of vitreous immune and biomarkers. In: Tsin A, editor. Early Events in Diabetic Retinopathy and Intervention Strategies Andrew Tsin. IntechOpen; 2018. pp. 71-91. DOI: 10.5772/intechopen.74366. Available from: https://www.intechopen.com/books/early-events-in-diabetic-retinopathy-and-intervention-strategies/proliferative-diabetic-retinopathy-an-overview-of-vitreous-immune-and-biomarkers

[24] Catanzaro OL, Capponi JA, Di Martino I, Labal ES, Sirois P. Oxidative stress in the optic nerve and visual area of steptozocin-induced diabetic Wistar rats: Blockade with selective bradykinin B1 receptor antagonist. Neuropeptides. 2017;**66**:97-102. DOI: 10.1016/j.npep.2017.10.003

[25] Kadłubowska J, Malaguarnera L, Wąż P, Zorena K. Neurodegeneration and neuroinflammation in diabetic retinopathy: Potential approaches to delay neuronal loss. Current Neuropharmacology. 2015;**14**:831-839. DOI: 10.2174/1570159X14666160614095559

[26] Yu Y, Chen H, Su SB. Neuroinflammatory responses in diabetic retinopathy. Journal of Neuroinflammation. 2015;**12**:141. DOI: 10.1186/s12974-015-0368-7

[27] Amano S, Kaji Y, Oshika T, Oka T, Machinami R, Nagai R, et al. Advanced glycation end products in human optic nerve head. The British Journal of Ophthalmology. 2001; **85**:52-55

[28] Madsen-Bouterse SA, Kowluru RA. Oxidative stress and diabetic retinopathy: Patho physiological mechanisms and treatment perspectives. Reviews in Endocrine & Metabolic Disorders. 2008;**9**(4):315-327. DOI: 10.1007/s11154-008-9090-4

[29] Simó R, Hernández C. Neurodegeneration in the diabetic eye: New insights and therapeutic perspectives. Trends in Endocrinology and Metabolism. 2014;**25**(1):23-33. DOI: 10.1016/j.tem.2013.09.005

[30] Xiao C, He M, Nan Y, Zhang D, Chen B, Guan Y, et al. Physiological effects of superoxide dismutase on altered visual function of retinal ganglion cells in db/db mice. PLoS One. 2012;**7**(1):e30343. DOI: 10.1371/journal.pone.0030343

[31] Fukumoto M, Nakaizumi A, Zhang T, Lentz SI, Shibata M, Puro DG. Vulnerability of the retinal microvasculature to oxidative stress: Ion channel-dependent mechanisms. American Journal of Physiology. Cell Physiology. 2012;**302**(9):C1413-C1420. DOI: 10.1152/ajpcell.00426.2011

[32] Li Q, Puro DG. Diabetes-induced dysfunction of the glutamate transporter in Müller cells. Investigative Ophthalmology & Visual Science. 2002;**43**(9):3109-3116

[33] Ng YK, Zeng XX, Ling EA. Expression of glutamate receptors and calcium-binding proteins in the retina of streptozotocin-induced diabetic rats. Brain Research. 2004;**1018**(1): 66-72. DOI: 10.1016/j.brainres.2004.05.055

[34] Santiago AR, Gaspar JM, Baptista FI, Cristóvão AJ, Santos PF, Kamphuis W, et al. Diabetes changes the level of ionotropic glutamate receptors in the rat retina. Molecular Vision. 2009;**15**:1620-1630

[35] Kaur C, Foulds WS, Ling EA. Hypoxia-ischemia and retinal ganglion cell damage. Clinical Ophthalmology. 2008;**2**(4):879-889

[36] Zhang L et al. Alterations in retrograde axonal transport in optic nerve of type I and type II diabetic rats. The Kobe Journal of Medical Sciences. 1998;**44**:205-215. [PubMed: 10401224]

[37] Fernandez DC et al. Early distal axonopathy of the visual pathway in experimental diabetes. The American Journal of Pathology. 2012;**180**:303-313. DOI: 310.1016/j.ajpath.2011.1009.1018. Epub 2011 Nov 1010. [PubMed: 22079928]

[38] Sokol S, Moskowitz A, Skarf B. Contrast sensitivity in diabetics with and without background retinopathy. Archives of Ophthalmology. 1985;**103**(1):51-54

[39] Katz G, Levkovitch-Verbin H, Treister G, et al. Mesopic foveal contrast sensitivity is impaired in diabetic patients without retinopathy. Graefe's Archive for Clinical and Experimental Ophthalmology. 2010;**248**(12):1699-1703

[40] Racette L, Sample PA. Short-wavelength automated perimetry. Ophthalmology Clinics of North America. 2003;**16**:227-236. vi-vii

[41] Lynch SK, Abràmoff MD. Diabetic retinopathy is a neurodegenerative disorder. Vision Research. 2017;**139**(2017):101-107. DOI: 10.1016/j.visres.2017.03.003

[42] Peduzzi M, Melli M, Fonda S, Codeluppi L, Guerrieri F. Comparative evaluation of blood viscosity in diabetic retinopathy. International Ophthalmology. 1984;**7**(1):15-19

[43] Rimmer T, Fleming J, Kohner EM. Hypoxic viscosity and diabetic retinopathy. British Journal of Ophthalmology. 1990;**74**:400-404

[44] Victor AA, Gondhowiardjo TD, Waspadji S, Wanandi SI, Bachtiar A, Suyatna FD, et al. Effect of laser photocoagulation and bevacizumab intravitreal in proliferative diabetic retinopathy: Review on biomarkers of oxidative stress. Medical Journal of Indonesia. 2014;**23**(2):79-86

[45] Bandello F, Rosangela L, Zucchiatti I, Del Turco C. Pathophysiology and treatment of diabetic retinopathy. Acta Diabetologica. 2013;**50**(1):1-20

[46] Antonetti DA, Klein R, Gardner TW. Mechanisms of disease diabetic retinopathy. The New England Journal of Medicine. 2012;**366**:1227-1239

[47] Tarr JM, Kaul K, Chopra M, Kohner EM, Chibber R. Pathophysiology of diabetic retino pathy. ISRN Ophthalmology. 2013;**2012**:1-13

[48] Ghanchi F, Bailey C, Chakravarthy U, Cohen S, Dodson P, Gibson J, et al. Diabetic Retino pathy Guidelines. London: The Royal College of Ophthalmologists; 2012. pp. 9-64

[49] Sayin N, Kara N, Pekel G. Ocular complications of diabetes mellitus. World Journal of Diabetes. 2015;**6**(1):92-108. DOI: 10.4239/wjd.v6.i1.92

[50] Slagle WS, Musick AN, Eckermann DR. Diabetic papillopathy and its relation to optic nerve ischemia. Optometry and Vision Science. 2009;**86**:E395-E403. DOI: 1040-5488/09/ 8604-0395/0

[51] Giuliari GP, Sadaka A, Chang PY, Cortez RT. Diabetic papillopathy: Current and new treatment options. Current Diabetes Reviews. 2011;**7**(3):171-175

[52] Barbera LG, Weiss MJ, Hofeldt AJ. Diabetic retinopathy and diabetic papillopathy. Seminars in Neurology. 1996;**16**(2):179-185

[53] Ciulla TA, Amador AG, Zinman B. Diabetic retinopathy and diabetic macular edema: Pathophysiology, screening, and novel therapies. Diabetes Care. 2003;**26**:2653-2664

[54] Bayraktar Z, Alacali N, Bayraktar S. Diabetic papillopathy in type II diabetic patients. Retina. 2002;**22**:752-758

[55] Hayreh SS, Zimmerman MB. Nonarteritic anterior ischemic optic neuropathy: Clinical characteristics in diabetic patients versus nondiabetic patients. Ophthalmology. 2008; **115**:1818-1825

[56] Brancato R, Menchini U, Bandello FM. Diabetic papillopathy: Fluorangiographic aspects. Metabolic, Pediatric, and Systemic Ophthalmology. 1986;**9**:57-61

[57] Regillo CD, Brown GC, Savino PJ, Byrnes GA, Benson WE, Tasman WS, et al. Diabetic papillopathy: Patient characteristics and fundus findings. Archives of Ophthalmology. 1995;**113**:889-895

[58] Shin SY, Kim DS, Ko MK. Fluorescein angiographic features of choroidal insufficiency in anterior ischemic optic neuropathy. Korean Journal of Ophthalmology. 1999;**13**:100-104

[59] Ostri C, Lund-Andersen H, Sander B, Hvidt-Nielsen D, Larsen M. Bilateral diabetic papillopathy and metabolic control. Ophthalmology. 2010;**117**:2214-2217. DOI: 10.1016/j. ophtha.2010.03.006

[60] Lubow M, Makley T. Pseudopapilledema of juvenile diabetes mellitus. Archives of Oph-thalmology. 2007;**85**:417-422

[61] Appen RE, Chandra SR, Klein R, Myers FL. Diabetic papillopathy. American Journal of Ophthalmology. 1980;**90**:203-209

[62] Freund M, Carmon A, Cohen AM. Papilledema and papillitis in diabetes: Report of two cases. American Journal of Ophthalmology. 1965;**60**:18-20

[63] Ciulla TA, Harris A, Latkany P, Piper HC, Arend O, Garzozi H, et al. Ocular perfusion abnormalities in diabetes. Acta Ophthalmologica Scandinavica. 2002;**80**:468-477

[64] Yanko L, Ticho U, Ivry M. Optic nerve involvement in diabetes. Acta Ophthalmologica. 1972;**50**:556-564

[65] Kim M, Lee JH, Lee SJ. Diabetic papillopathy with macular edema treated with intravitreal ranibizumab. Clinical Ophthalmology. 2013;**7**:2257-2260

[66] Al-Hinai AS, Al-Abri MS, Al-Hajri RH. Diabetic papillopathy with macular edema treated with intravitreal bevacizumab. Oman Journal of Ophthalmology. 2011;**4**:135-138

[67] Al-Dhibi H, Khan AO. Response of diabetic papillopathy to intravitreal bevacizumab. Middle East African Journal of Ophthalmology. 2011;**18**:243-245

[68] Willerslev A, Munch IC, Larsen M. Resolution of diabetic papillopathy after a single intravitreal injection of ranibizumab. Acta Ophthalmologica. 2012;**90**:e407-e409

[69] Mansour AM, El-Dairi MA, Shehab MA, Shahin HK, Shaaban JA, Antonios SR. Periocular corticosteroids in diabetic papillopathy. Eye (London, England). 2005;**19**:45-51

[70] Yassur Y, Pickle LW, Fine SL, Singerman L, Orth DH, Patz A. Optic disc neovascularisation in diabetic retinopathy: A system for grading proliferation at the optic nerve head in patients with proliferative diabetic retinopathy. British Journal of Ophthalmology. 1980;**64**:69-76

[71] Jeganathan VSE, Wardrop D. A paradigm shift in the management of neovascular glaucoma. New Frontiers in Ophthalmology. 2016;**2**(3):119-124. DOI: 10.15761/NFO.1000128

[72] Jeganathan VSE, Wang JJ, Wong TY. Ocular associations of diabetes other than diabetic retinopathy. Diabetes Care. 2008;**31**(9):1905-1912. DOI: 10.2337/dc08-0342

[73] Rodrigues GB, Abe RY, Zangalli C, Sodre SL, Donini FA, Costa DC, et al. Neovascular glaucoma: A review. International Journal of Retina and Vitreous. 2016;**2**:26. DOI: 10.1186/s40942-016-0051-x

[74] Hayreh SS. Neovascular glaucoma. Progress in Retinal and Eye Research. 2007;**26**:470-485

[75] Akiyama H, Li D, Shimoda Y, Matsumoto H, Kishi S. Observation of neovascularization of the disc associated with proliferative diabetic retinopathy using OCT angiography. Japanese Journal of Ophthalmology. 2018;**62**(3):286-291. DOI: 10.1007/s10384-018-0571-z

[76] Dubey S, Pegu J. Management of neovascular glaucoma. Journal of Current Glaucoma Practice. 2009;**3**(3):27-34

[77] Venkatramani DV, Amula GM, Gandhi RA. Optic Atrophy. Kerala Journal of Ophthalmology. 2010;**22**(1):7-12

[78] Gandhi R, Amula GA. Optic Atrophy. Medscape. 2016. Available from: https://emedicine.medscape.com/article/1217760-overview#a4

[79] Adachi M, Takahashi K, Nishikawa M, Miki H, Uyama M. High intraocular pressure-induced ischemia and reperfusion injury in the optic nerve and retina in rats. Graefe's

Archive for Clinical and Experimental Ophthalmology. 1996;**234**:445-451. DOI: 10.1007/bf02539411

[80] Joachim SC, Wax MB, Boehm N, Dirk DR, Pfeiffer N, Grus FH. Upregulation of antibody response to heat shock proteins and tissue antigens in an ocular ischemia model. Investigative Ophthalmology & Visual Science. 2011;**52**:3468-3474. DOI: 10.1167/iovs.10-5763

[81] Renner M, Stute G, Alzureiqi M, Reinhard J, Wiemann S, Schmid H, et al. Optic nerve degeneration after retinal ischemia/reperfusion in a rodent model. Frontiers in Cellular Neuroscience. 2017;**11**:254. DOI: 10.3389/fncel.2017.00254

[82] Safi H, Safi S, Hafezi-Moghadam A, Ahmadieh H. Early Detection of Diabetic Retinopathy. Survey of Ophthalmology. 2018;**63**(5):601-608. DOI: 10.1016/j.survophthal.2018.04.003

[83] Anderson AJ, Johnson CA. Mechanisms isolated by frequencydoubling technology perimetry. Investigative Ophthalmology & Visual Science. 2002;**43**:398-401

[84] Frisen L. New, sensitive window on abnormal spatial vision: Rarebit probing. Vision Research. 2002;**42**:1931-1939

[85] Bengtsson B, Heijl A, Agardh E. Visual fields correlate better than visual acuity to severity of diabetic retinopathy. Diabetologia. 2005;**48**:2494-2500

[86] Kumar KVSH, Ahmad FMH, Sood S, Mansingh S. Visual evoked potential to assess retinopathy in gestational diabetes mellitus. Canadian Journal of Diabetes. 2015:1-4

[87] Nasralah Z, Robinson W, Jackson GR, Barber AJ. Measuring visual function in diabetic retinopathy: Progress in basic and clinical research. Journal of Clinical and Experimental Ophthalmology. 2013;**4**:306. DOI: 10.4172/2155-9570.1000306

[88] Shankar U, Gunasundari R. A review on electrophysiology based detection of diabetic retinopathy. Procedia Computer Science. 2015;**48**:630-637

[89] Kumar R, Sundararajan D, Ponraj RS, Srinivasan M. A study on early detection of changes in visual pathway due to diabetes mellitus by visual evoked potential. International Journal of Medical Research and Health Sciences. 2014;**3**(1):161-164

[90] Vujosevic S, Simo R. Local and systemic inflammatory biomarkers of diabetic retinopathy: An integrative approach. Investigative Ophthalmology & Visual Science. 2017;**58**(6): Bio68-bio75

[91] Kaviarasan K, Jithu M, Arif Mulla M, et al. Low blood and vitreal BDNF, LXA4 and altered Th1/Th2 cytokine balance are potential risk factors for diabetic retinopathy. Metabolism. 2015;**64**(9):958-966

[92] Demirkaya N, van-Dijk HW, van-Schuppen SM, Abràmoff MD, Garvin MK, Sonka M, et al. Effect of age on individual retinal layer thickness in normal eyes as measured with spectral-domain optical coherence tomography. Investigative Ophthalmology and Visual Science. 2013;**54**(7):4934-4940

[93] Tawse KL, Hedges TR, Gobuty M, Mendoza-Santiesteban C. Optical coherence tomography shows retinal abnormalities associated with optic nerve disease. Brazilian Journal of Ophthalmology. 2014;**98**(Suppl 2):ii30-ii33. DOI: 10.1136/bjophthalmol-2013-304301

[94] Lamirel C, Newman NJ, Biousse V. Optical coherence tomography (OCT) in optic neuritis and multiple sclerosis. Revista de Neurologia. 2010;**166**(12):978-986. DOI: 10.1016/j.neurol.2010.03.024

[95] Ishibazawa A, Nagaoka T, Yokota H, Takahashi A, Omae T, Song Y, et al. Characteristics of retinal neovascularization in proliferative diabetic retinopathy imaged by optical coherence tomography angiography. Investigative Ophthalmology & Visual Science. 2016;**57**:6247-6255. DOI: 10.1167/iovs.16-20210

[96] Savastano MC, Federici M, Falsini B, Caporossi A, Minnella AM. Detecting papillary neovascularization inproliferative diabetic retinopathy using opticalcoherence tomography angiography. Acta Ophthalmologica. 2018;**96**(3):321-323. DOI: 10.1111/aos.13166

Section 2

Clinical Challenges in Optic Nerve Disorder Management

Chapter 5

Evaluation of Retinal Nerve Fiber Layer and Inner Macular Layers in Primary Open-Angle Glaucoma with Spectral-Domain Optical Coherence Tomography

Bilyana Mihaylova and Galina Dimitrova

Additional information is available at the end of the chapter

http://dx.doi.org/10.5772/intechopen.79102

Abstract

The aim of our research is to assess and compare the peripapillary retinal nerve fiber layer (pRNFL) thickness diagnostic capability with those of three macular parameters—macular RNFL (mRNFL) thickness, GCL+ (ganglion cell layer with inner plexiform layer thickness), and GCL++ (mRNFL and GCL+) in primary open-angle glaucoma patients with spectral-domain optical coherence tomography (SD-OCT).

The 414 participants (483 eyes) aged 45–84 years in this prospective study were recruited from Eye Clinic at the University Hospital "Alexandrovska" (Sofia, Bulgaria). They were divided into 6 groups: controls, ocular hypertension, preperimetric glaucoma (PPG), and three groups of perimetric glaucoma stages—early, moderate, and advanced. OCT was performed using Topcon 3D OCT 2000 device, as eight parameters from two protocols (Circle and Glaucoma Analysis—Macula) were analyzed. The results showed that the RNFL highest diagnostic capability parameter is Total mRNFL (AUROC 0.879 in PPG and 0.929 in early glaucoma stage). The macular highest diagnostic accuracy parameter was found GCL++ without any significance from mRNFL diagnostic possibilities.

The results of current research showed that mRNFL possesses high diagnostic accuracy in comparison analysis with other pRNFL and macular OCT parameters in early glaucomatous changes. Macular RNFL and its highest diagnostic possibilities could be successfully used as an individual diagnostic parameter separated from the whole ganglion cell complex in the early glaucoma changes.

Keywords: primary open-angle glaucoma, retinal nerve fiber layer, inner macular layers, optical coherence tomography

1. Introduction

According to the American Academy of Ophthalmology the medical term glaucoma is used for a group of diseases that damage the optic nerve (ON) as distinctive type of optic neuropathy characterized by structural (cupping of optic nerve head—ONH, changes in connective tissue structural elements and number of the nerve fibers in ON) and functional changes (typical visual field defects). Increased intraocular pressure (IOP) is one of the most common risk factors associated with developing and progressing of the disease, but its presence or absence does not change the above-mentioned glaucoma definition [1].

Epidemiological studies found that the glaucoma at the end of twentieth century covered more than 60 million people around the world. Prognostic studies show an increasing trend of the number of affected patients, and in 2020 it is going to be approximately 80 million people, and in 2040 approximately 112 million [2–4]. Cataract and glaucoma are leading causes of blindness worldwide. Because of the reversibility of the vision after cataract extraction, the glaucoma remains the leading cause of irreversible blindness. The large number of glaucoma patients, irreversible vision loss and the impact on the life quality of the affected people are just part of the reasons for making glaucoma one of the diseases with big social influence.

Glaucoma is characterized by irreversible loss of ganglion cells, which axons form the ON. Ganglion cells are localized in three retinal layers—inner plexiform layer or IPL (their dendrites), ganglion cell layer or GCL (their bodies), and retinal nerve fiber layer or RNFL (their axons). Therefore exactly the above-mentioned layers are those, which glaucoma affects accompanying typical visual field defects [5]. Chronic and progressive loss of neuroretinal tissue is cardinal feature of glaucomatous optic neuropathy (GON) and criterion for diagnosis [6].

1.1. Anatomical aspects of the RNFL

All afferent pathways in the ON start from a layer of photoreceptors (cones and rods), which is located in the retina on area more than 1000 mm^2. In ONH all fibers are concentrated on surface with approximately 2–3 mm^2 area [7, 8]. From the body of each ganglion cell comes out a nerve fiber or axon, which moves toward the ONH. So that it can be called conglomerate consisted of all converging axons, which are as mentioned above part of the retina and form a layer—RNFL [9]. Nowhere else the ganglions' nerve fibers are not so much compact as they are in ONH, and this is what determines the importance of peripapillary RNFL thickness in diagnosis and follow up of patients with GON.

These are some characteristics of RNFL [9, 10]:

1. Papillomacular nerve fiber bundle—it starts from ganglion cells in the foveolar region. The nerve fibers from nasal foveolar area move straight toward the temporal border of ONH, and those from the temporal part make a slight arc around the nasal nerve fibers and then join to the straight bundle.

2. Superior and inferior retinal arcades—they are created by later formed nerve fibers and ganglion cells originating temporal to the fovea. They arc around the macula and papillomacular bundle to enter the ONH.

3. Temporal raphe or seam—it extends from the fovea to the temporal part of the retina and consists of very few axons, because by rule the nerve fibers from the upper half of the retina do not pass the horizontal meridian to the arcuate course of the nerve fibers from the lower part of the retina, and vice versa.
4. An extremely large collection of nerve fibers in the superior and inferior quadrant of the ONH—namely these two regions are set to be more vulnerable for glaucomatous damages.
5. Nasal nerve fibers—they move radially toward the ONH.
6. Exact location of the nerve fibers in the ONH according to their position in the fundus—the more peripheral retinal location the more central ONH localization.

Basic features, used to make an assessment of RNFL images [9]:

1. Striations of RNFL—normally RNFL can be seen as striated bright and dark lines in the areas of superior and inferior temporal blood vessels in healthy eyes. If atrophy is presented (<50 μm RNFL thickness) the striations of the background disappear and bright lines cannot be seen because of the RNFL loss [11] (see **Figure 1**).
2. Defects of the background brightness—they can be diffuse loss and localized defects (wedge-shaped and cleft-shaped). The width in the cleft-shaped defects is the same along the full length, however the width in wedge-shaped defects is different, peripherally they are wider and become narrower toward the ONH. This could be explained with convergent course of the nerve fibers. Diffuse defects have an impact over the complete RNFL thickness in the fundus and also their diagnosis is more difficult from localized defects.
3. Visualization of the blood vessels—normally RNFL covers retinal blood vessels. That's why small and medium-sized blood vessels have unclear contours and look misty. When RNFL atrophy appears, then blood vessels can be seen clearly because of the less covering from the nerve fiber layer.

All nerve fibers are arranged in a specific way in the ONH not only in each and every human being but also in each and every of the human eyes. Equal quantity nerve fibers may look in a different way in the borders of ONHs with dissimilar disc area, depth of the lamina cribrosa, and height of the scleral canal [12]. Equal functional capacitate could be presented by different looking structures and vice versa—equal looking structures could have different functional activity [13–15].

The RNFL thickness depends on: age, ethnicity, number and thickness of the nerve fibers, quantity of the glia, quantity of the blood vessels, disk area of the ONH, axial length of the eye (Ax). The thickness of the measured RNFL depends also on: the stage of peripapillary atrophy/conus myopicus, vitreoretinal tractions. The excavation (cupping) depends on: disc area, number and thickness of the nerve fibers, quantity of the glia [14]. Normally in the course of time the RNFL thickness decreases with age normally with 4000–5000 axons per year [16–19] and this is approximately 2.0 μm/decade or 0.2% per year at mean thickness 100 μm [20]. The ON consists of 700,000–1.4 million nerve fibers and the RNFL thickness in healthy people has a wide variety of a norm. The usage of absolute values restricts the process of distinguishing

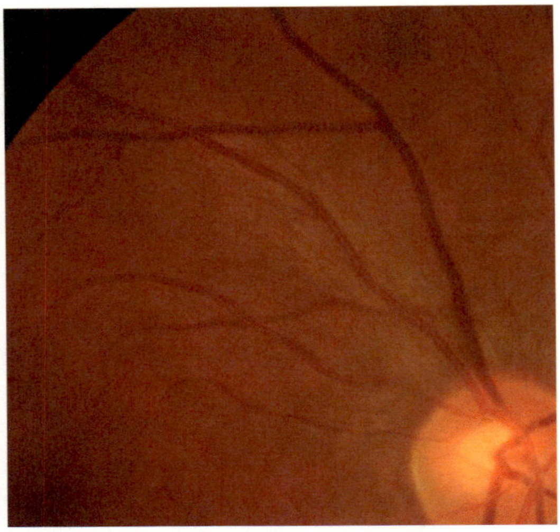

Figure 1. RNFL striations in superior temporal area of the fundus in healthy eye of 52 years old female.

healthy from glaucoma patients [20]. Therefore some authors talk about "modulation of RNFL thickness"—it shows the relative loss of nerve fibers as difference between the biggest and smallest measured value of RNFL thickness in a retinal region of interest [21].

1.2. RNFL and glaucoma

When assessing glaucomatous damages it is appropriate to measure the RNFL thickness, because thinning of this layer correlated directly with ganglion cells loss, which is the basic pathophysiological event [22]. Evaluation of the RNFL thickness is important for early glaucoma diagnosis before appearing of the clinical manifestations of the disease. It is proven that 40–50% of the nerve fibers are should be dropped out before developing of the visual field defects [23]. Clinical evaluation of the RNFL with red-free photography shows that thinning of the layer can be seen in 60% of the pictures 6 years before appearing of clinical manifestation of the defects in visual field [24]. These facts show that structural changes occur before the functional ones. Typical visual field defects in glaucoma are nasal step, arcuate scotoma, paracentral scotoma, generalized depression, and progressive worsening of the indices of the standard automated perimetry (SAP) [25].

Sometimes in glaucoma visual field defects can be seen without appearance of structural glaucomatous changes. It is possible also in equal RNFL loss to be obtained a different clinical finding according to initial RNFL thickness. This could be explained with the following: visual field defects appear after 40% loss of the nerve fibers. Each man is born with different quantity nerve fibers. If a person owns very thick for human population RNFL, the loss of 40% nerve fibers probably will not give any significant results in optical coherence tomography (OCT)—the line thickness will be in the middle of the green zone, the zone shows lack of disease. Then this individual is going to have functional defects with normal RNFL thickness. If another person is born with thin RNFL, the loss of 40% nerve fibers will give significant results—OCT line thickness will be close to the yellow zone or in the zone. Then this individual is going to have functional defects with pathological thin RNFL [14, 15].

In the early glaucoma stage it is considered that the affected ganglion cells decrease their functional processes before they die and this leads to decreasing of the visual functions without an obvious structural changes. This is the reason why a patient has functional manifestations of glaucoma in combination with normal RNFL thickness [14].

The most distant nerve fibers from ONH originate exactly from these farthest parts of the ganglion cells in the retina and they are located deeply in the RNFL. They pass closely to the scleral edge and most peripherally in the ON [26]. These nerve fibers that originate from the closest to the ONH parts of the retina are located superficially in the RNFL and pass centrally in the ON. It is thought that the nerve fibers, which are located superficially in the RNFL, are more vulnerable in glaucoma, and their damage is associated with an enlargement of the blind spot.

It is also believed that chronically increased IOP leads to compression of the circulation of the Elschnig's border tissue and its atrophy. Then lamina cribrosa starts posteriorization. It is considered therefore that it is a reason for stretching and rupturing of the nerve fibers which are closest to the scleral edge. Only nerve fibers in prelaminar region can drop out consequently, because they are separated and not in bundles. The affecting of the nerve fibers is from peripheral to central region [26, 27]. Unordered affecting of the nerve fibers can be seen in acute angle closure glaucoma.

2. Retinal nerve fiber layer and inner macular layers evaluation in primary open-angle glaucoma with spectral-domain optical coherence tomography

2.1. Purpose

The aim of our research is to assess and compare the peripapillary RNFL (pRNFL) thickness diagnostic capability with those of three macular parameters—macular RNFL (mRNFL) thickness, GCL+ (ganglion cell layer with inner plexiform layer thickness), and GCL++ (mRNFL and GCL+) in primary open-angle glaucoma patients with spectral-domain OCT (SD-OCT).

2.2. Material and methods

2.2.1. Material

All participants (healthy volunteers and patients) included in current clinical study were examined in the university eye clinic of Alexandrovska Hospital, Sofia, Bulgaria for total period of time—a year and 3 months. This is a prospective observational study of 414 participants (483 eyes) aged 45–84 years (mean 66.7 ± 8.7), male—132, and female—282. All patients were distributed into six groups:

I[st] group (**Controls**)—150 eyes, 150 healthy volunteers, mean age 63.0 ± 9.

IInd group (**Ocular hypertension** (OH))—50 eyes, 31 patients, mean age 60.1 ± 9.2.

IIIrd group (**Preperimetric glaucoma** (PPG))—62 eyes, 49 patients, mean age 66.3 ± 7.5.

IVth group (**Early perimetric POAG**)—96 eyes, 80 patients, mean age 69.7 ± 7.9.

V[th] group (**Moderate perimetric POAG**)—40 eyes, 34 patients, mean age 70.4 ± 8.5.

VIth group (**Advanced perimetric POAG**)—85 eyes, 70 patients, mean age 69.5 ± 9.8.

The following inclusion and exclusion criteria were defined for the groups:

Inclusion criteria for the control group: healthy participants without congenital or acquired general or eye diseases exception of early age-related cataract; people without family history and other risk factors for glaucoma; best corrected visual acuity (BCVA) = 1.0; refraction error in ±4.00 dsph and ±1.00 dcyl; IOP under 21 mmHg measured with Goldmann tonometer according to central corneal thickness (CCT) values; open anterior chamber angle class III–IV Shaffer Angle Classification System; ocular fundus without glaucomatous damages—vital optic nerve head (ONH), ISNT rule in norm, C/D Ratio < 0.5 PD and interocular asymmetry in C/D Ratio ≤ 0.2 PD; normal SAP (Glaucoma Hemifield Test—within normal limits, $p > 0.05$ for MD and PSD indices).

Inclusion criteria for OH group: patients with OH and any other coexisting ocular and general pathology; BCVA = 1.0; refraction error in ±4.00 dsph and ±1.00 dcyl; permanent elevation of IOP more than 21 mmHg measured with Goldmann tonometer without treatment and corrected according to the CCT values and daytime pressure curves; open anterior chamber angle; lack of pathological changes in the fundus; normal SAP.

Inclusion criteria for Preperimetric glaucoma group: BCVA = 1.0; refraction error in already shown limits; permanent elevation of IOP more than 21 mmHg; open anterior chamber angle; fundus glaucomatous changes: interocular asymmetry in C/D Ratio ≥ 0.2 PD, vertical elongated excavation, thinning of optic disc rim, local thinning of neuroretinal rim, violated ISNT rule, defects in RNFL thickness (diffuse or local), normal SAP.

Inclusion criteria for perimetric glaucoma groups: BCVA = 1.0 for early stage glaucoma group and BCVA ≥ 0.2 for moderate and advanced stage of POAG; refraction error in already shown limits; permanent elevation of IOP more than 21 mmHg; open anterior chamber angle; fundus glaucomatous changes: interocular asymmetry in C/D Ratio ≥ 0.2 PD, vertical elongated excavation, thinning of optic disc rim, local thinning of neuroretinal rim, violated ISNT rule, defects in RNFL thickness (diffuse or local), ONH hemorrhages; typical for glaucoma visual field defects in SAP corresponding with changes in ONH; glaucoma perimetric stage was defined as changes in SAP based on Hodapp-Parrish-Anderson classification.

Exclusion criteria: best corrected visual acuity ≤ 0.2; age < 45 years and > 85 years; refraction error beyond already shown limits; normotensive glaucoma, angle closure glaucoma; macular pathology, diabetic retinopathy, nonglaucomatous opticopathy; previous eye surgery (exception cataract refractive surgery with intraocular lens implantation); coexisting neurological pathology which can influence on the visual field results.

2.2.2. Methods

All patients underwent full ophthalmological examination including: a complete case history for eye and general diseases; family history; refraction and best corrected visual acuity; slit-lamp examination; indirect fundus biomicroscopy; contact ultrasound pachymetry (OcuScan RxP - Alcon, Forth Worth, Texas, USA); Goldmann tonometry; indirect gonioscopy (Goldmann three-mirror gonioprism/Shaffer classification, 1960); SAP - SITA Standard 24-2, HFA II (Carl Zeiss Meditec, Dublin, CA, USA) with near correction if necessary. Only reliable perimetry results with total error rate (loss of fixation and false-positive and false-negative results) lower than 25%. The stage of POAG changes was determined using Hodapp-Parrish-Anderson classification.

Optical coherence tomography: All patients underwent SD-OCT of both eyes with dilated pupils by one examiner using Topcon 3D OCT 2000 (FA plus) (Topcon Corporation, Japan), software version - 8.11.

The following programs were used:

- Circle program evaluated peripapillary RNFL thickness. From Circle protocol we analyzed the following parameters: (1) Total pRNFL—showed the average thickness in 360°; (2) Sup pRNFL—showed the thickness in the superior 90°; (3) Inf pRNFL—showed the thickness in the inferior 90°; (4) Nas pRNFL—showed the thickness in the nasal 90°; (5) Temp pRNFL—showed the thickness in the temporal 90° (see **Figure 2**, right).
- 3D Macula (V) program is used for the internal macular layers thickness evaluation in area of 7 mm^2. The following parameters were analyzed: (1) Sup mRNFL (Sup mRNFL)—mRNFL thickness in the upper half; (2) Inf mRNFL (Inf mRNFL)—in the lower half; (3) Total mRNFL (Total mRNFL)—in the whole macular area (see **Figure 2**, left).

Only OCT protocols with scan quality over 50%, no artifacts from eye or body movements, blinking, and lack of macular pathology (edema, drusen, holes) were included in the analysis.

Statistical methods: For statistically significant were considered the differences with P values <0.05. We used descriptive, dispersion and ROC-analysis to evaluate diagnostic accuracy, specificity, and sensitivity. A comparison was made between Ist group and IInd, Ist and IIIrd and so long. With comparison analysis we searched for statistical significant difference between some of the parameters' values in specificity and sensitivity.

2.3. Results

The descriptive statistics can be seen in **Table 1**, and mean values of the all RNFL parameters in **Table 2**. In **Table 3** can be seen the ROC analysis and the diagnostic capabilities of the eight OCT parameters in each group. The RNFL parameter with highest diagnostic potential in the groups—PPG (AUROC = 0.879), early (AUROC = 0.929), moderate (AUROC = 0.989) and advanced glaucoma (AUROC = 1.000) is Total mRNFL followed by Inf mRNFL and Inf pRNFL. The RNFL parameters with lowest diagnostic potential in all glaucoma stages are Nas pRNFL, Temp RNFL. A single RNFL parameter (Total mRNFL) was measured with

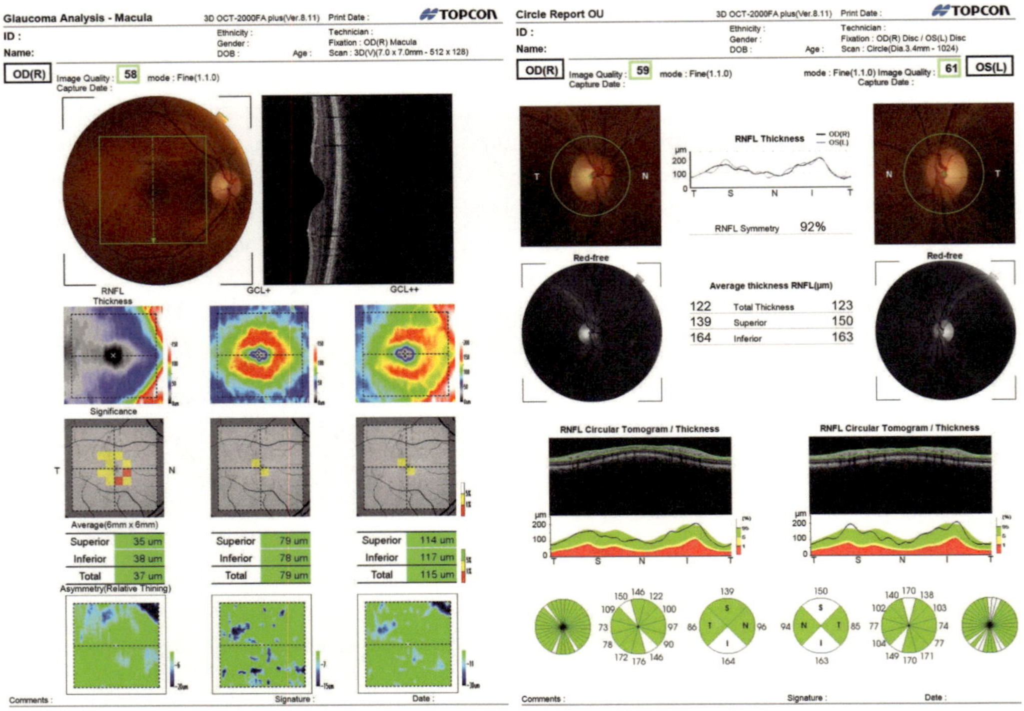

Figure 2. Glaucoma analysis—Macula protocol (left) and Circle protocol (right).

highest diagnostic accuracy for glaucoma in all of its stages - from PPG to advanced glaucoma. In the current investigation, it is shown for the first time the higher diagnostic ability of macular RNFL from those of peripapillary RNFL. In OH group, we found that Inf mRNFL has the highest diagnostic possibilities but without any clinical significance, because none of the RNFL parameters change significantly in patients with OH in comparison with control group.

AUROC values allowed us to create ROC curves in all groups as we included the five RNFL parameters with the best results (**Figures 3–6**).

After that we used comparison analysis to demonstrate if statistical significant difference exists between diagnostic possibilities of RNFL parameters in all groups. In **Table 4** can be seen only two significant differences in AUROC values between Sup mRNFL (0.907) and Total mRNFL, and between Total mRNFL (0.929) and Inf pRNFL (0.867). Although, we found the highest diagnostic potential in all glaucoma groups for Total mRNFL, our comparison analysis showed that these possibilities are not statistical significant with exception of the above-mentioned two examples. For instance, in the stage of PPG, we were not able to find any statistical significant differences between the best five diagnostic RNFL parameters (**Table 4**), so they have equal abilities to diagnose glaucoma patients in this particular stage. In the stage of early POAG, we found significant difference in diagnostic abilities between Inf pRNFL and Total mRNFL, so that it would be better if the clinician uses not the first five but the four best diagnostic parameters from **Table 3**.

Group	Sex	Number	Age (years)			
			Mean	SD	Min	Max
Controls	Men—m	30	61.7	9.7	48.0	81.0
	Women—f	120	63.4	8.9	45.0	84.0
	All	150	63.0	9.0	45.0	84.0
OH	m	10	59.4	10.6	45.0	76.0
	f	21	60.4	8.6	45.0	72.0
	All	31	60.1	9.2	45.0	76.0
Preperimetric glaucoma	m	20	68.6	6.9	51.0	81.0
	f	29	64.7	7.6	45.0	74.0
	All	49	66.3	7.5	45.0	81.0
Early glaucoma	m	30	71.7	6.0	58.0	81.0
	f	50	68.5	8.7	45.0	82.0
	All	80	69.7	7.9	45.0	82.0
Moderate glaucoma	m	11	70.5	10.2	45.0	82.0
	f	23	70.4	7.9	57.0	81.0
	All	34	70.4	8.5	45.0	82.0
Advanced glaucoma	m	31	67.7	11.5	45.0	83.0
	f	39	70.7	8.2	45.0	84.0
	All	70	69.5	9.8	45.0	84.0

Table 1. Descriptive statistics.

We evaluated also sensitivity, specificity and cut-off values for the same RNFL parameters. In PPG group there are two parameters with highest and almost equal values of the sensitivity and specificity—Total mRNFL (sensitivity—0.83, specificity—0.77) and Inf mRNFL (sensitivity—0.82, specificity—0.79). These two parameters keep their high and close values of sensitivity also in the group of early perimetric glaucoma: Total mRNFL—0.93 и Inf mRNFL—0.90. The parameter with highest value of specificity in the same group is Total pRNFL—0.89, and after it are these parameters: Total mRNFL—0.81 and Inf mRNFL—0.79. In the PPG group with highest values is Total mRNFL (sensitivity—0.97 and specificity—0.95), and after it is Inf mRNFL (sensitivity—0.94 and specificity—0.85). It is observed very small differences in the values between investigated parameters, which decrease in advanced glaucoma group. With highest sensitivity (1.00) and specificity (1.00) in advanced glaucoma group is Total mRNFL, and after it is Inf pRNFL (1.00; 0.99) and Inf mRNFL (0.99, 0.99).

In **Table 5** can be seen the AUROC values of the macular parameters—Total mRNFL, Total GCL+ (ganglion cell layer/GCL + inner plexiform layer/IPL) and Total GCL++ (GCL + IPL + mRNFL) from protocol Glaucoma Analysis—Macula (see **Figure 3**, left). Lowest diagnostic

Parameter (μm)	Controls	OH	Preperimetric glaucoma	Early glaucoma	Moderate glaucoma	Advanced glaucoma
	Mean ± SD	**Mean ± SD**	**Mean ± SD**	**Mean ± SD**	**Mean ± SD**	**Mean ± SD**
MD [dB]	−0.24 ± 1.30	−0.05 ± 1.15	−0.60 ± 1.13	−2.73 ± 1.85	−8.65 ± 1.77	−21.44 ± 5.81
PSD [dB]	1.72 ± 0.38	1.59 ± 0.32	1.82 ± 0.33	3.72 ± 1.73	7.84 ± 2.66	9.26 ± 3.15
Sup mRNFL	36.09 ± 4.30	36.46 ± 5.77	30.58 ± 3.75	28.90 ± 4.90	24.60 ± 6.85	16.78 ± 6.58
Inf mRNFL	39.22 ± 5.27	38.16 ± 4.69	31.34 ± 5.01	29.44 ± 5.81	25.05 ± 7.04	14.20 ± 6.33
Total mRNFL	37.67 ± 4.23	37.30 ± 4.67	31.05 ± 4.06	29.21 ± 4.37	25.00 ± 4.75	15.48 ± 5.58
Sup pRNFL	122.31 ± 12.09	128.70 ± 14.86	111.34 ± 17.17	101.47 ± 14.18	90.38 ± 20.29	77.47 ± 16.26
Inf pRNFL	136.86 ± 14.46	137.66 ± 14.65	115.74 ± 18.14	108.05 ± 22.62	90.53 ± 23.59	69.22 ± 15.03
Nas pRNFL	90.55 ± 14.73	92.24 ± 18.47	81.98 ± 19.99	82.23 ± 18.00	74.58 ± 19.36	66.99 ± 16.63
Temp pRNFL	81.62 ± 11.76	85.92 ± 16.12	74.26 ± 14.88	72.98 ± 15.62	69.28 ± 17.88	60.35 ± 15.76
Total pRNFL	107.84 ± 7.95	111.14 ± 10.25	95.92 ± 12.26	90.81 ± 12.48	81.15 ± 15.28	68.46 ± 12.32

Table 2. Mean values and standard deviation (SD) of RNFL in all groups.

Parameter	OH	Preperimetric glaucoma	Early glaucoma	Moderate glaucoma	Advanced glaucoma
	AUROC	**AUROC**	**AUROC**	**AUROC**	**AUROC**
Sup pRNFL	0.364	0.694	0.866	0.903	0.983
Inf pRNFL	0.472	0.820	0.867	0.957	0.999
Nas pRNFL	0.486	0.627	0.643	0.731	0.874
Temp pRNFL	0.428	0.678	0.687	0.719	0.893
Total pRNFL	0.412	0.791	0.900	0.947	0.993
Sup mRNFL	0.514	0.839	0.886	0.907	0.996
Inf mRNFL	**0.563**	0.864	0.907	0.951	0.997
Total mRNFL	0.535	**0.879**	**0.929**	**0.989**	**1.000**

Table 3. ROC-analysis.

accuracy for glaucoma in all investigated stages possesses the parameter—GCL+. The highest area under the curve has GCL++ (0.919, 0.932) in PPG group, Total mRNFL in the moderate glaucoma group (0.989), and the both parameters reach maximal possibilities for diagnosis in advanced glaucoma group (1.000). We also applied comparison analysis to find significance in diagnostic capabilities (AUROC values) between macular parameters. The results from this analysis could be seen in **Table 6**. Significance can be seen in the values between Total mRNFL and Total GCL+, and between Total GCL++ and Total GCL+. We did not find a difference between Total mRNFL and Total GCL++. This mean that the whole ganglion cell

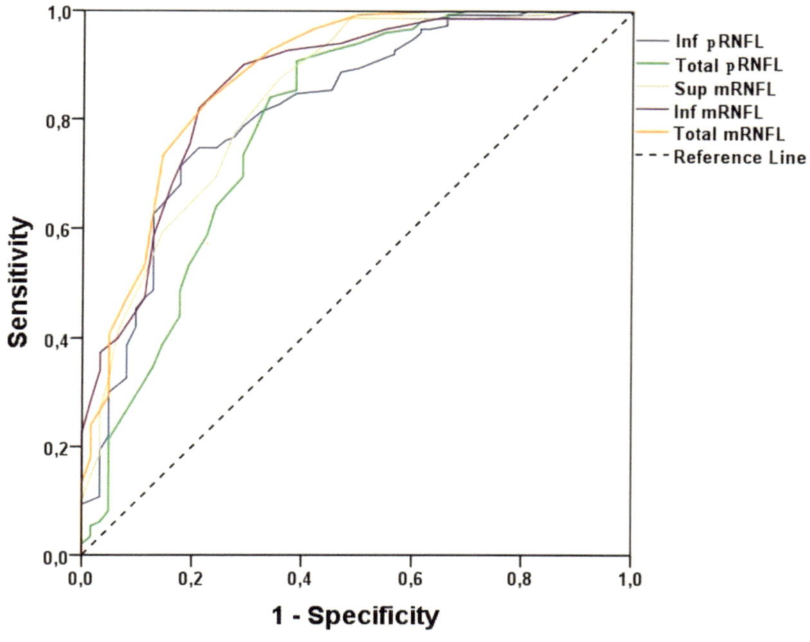

Figure 3. PPG.

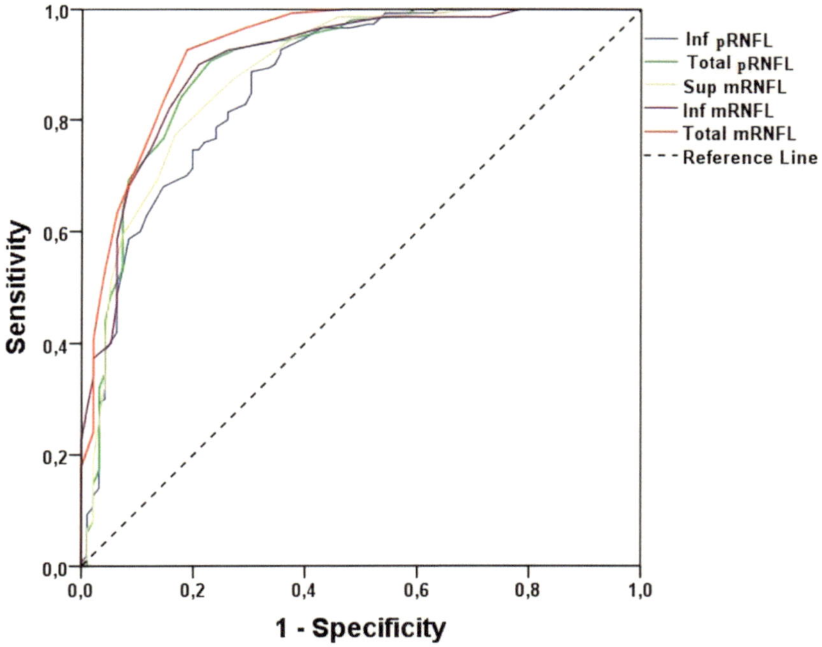

Figure 4. Early glaucoma.

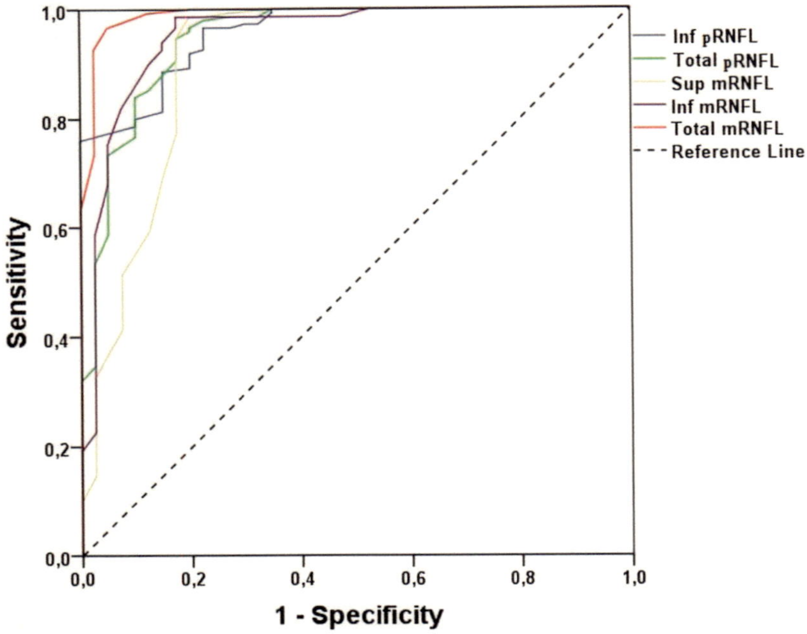

Figure 5. Moderate glaucoma.

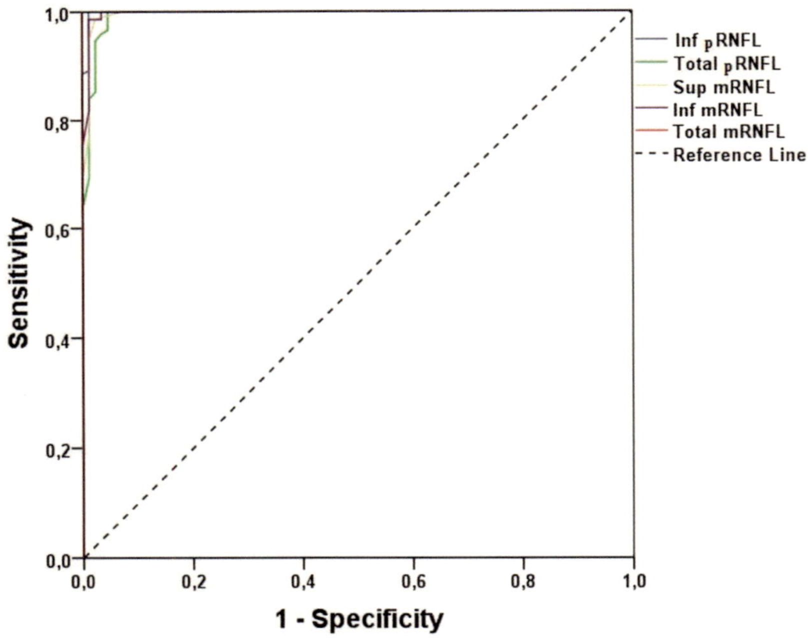

Figure 6. Advanced glaucoma.

http://dx.doi.org/10.5772/intechopen.79102

AUROC comparisons		Controls vs.			
		PPG	Early glaucoma	Moderate glaucoma	Advanced glaucoma
		p	p	p	p
Sup mRNFL	Inf mRNFL	0.587	0.486	0.280	0.806
Sup mRNFL	Total mRNFL	0.339	0.136	**0.019**	0.238
Sup mRNFL	Inf pRNFL	0.680	0.571	0.178	0.469
Sup mRNFL	Total pRNFL	0.329	0.673	0.327	0.603
Inf mRNFL	Total mRNFL	0.702	0.410	0.115	0.275
Inf mRNFL	Inf pRNFL	0.315	0.204	0.832	0.601
Inf mRNFL	Total pRNFL	0.125	0.796	0.884	0.451
Total mRNFL	Inf pRNFL	0.172	**0.041**	0.050	0.339
Total mRNFL	Total pRNFL	0.062	0.296	0.068	0.132
Inf pRNFL	Total pRNFL	0.558	0.326	0.694	0.245

Table 4. Comparison analysis in AUROC values in all groups.

Parameter	Controls vs.			
	PPG	Early glaucoma	Moderate glaucoma	Advanced glaucoma
	AUROC	AUROC	AUROC	AUROC
Total mRNFL	0.879	0.929	0.989	1.000
Total GCL+	0.839	0.858	0.939	0.993
Total GCL++	0.919	0.932	0.987	1.000

Table 5. AUROC values of the GCL map parameters.

layer (consists of three sub-layers), which is presented by GCL++ parameter, has an equivalent diagnostic potential of those of Total mRNFL, which presents only one of the macular sub-layers (the most inner layer consists of the nerve fibers). The less accurate diagnostic potential from macular OCT parameters we found for GCL++. Therefore we exclude this parameter as an accurate in glaucoma diagnosis.

2.4. Discussion

In the current research we found that the Topcon OCT parameter—Total mRNFL has the highest diagnostic accuracy in the very early stage of glaucoma, in which only structural changes could be seen (PPG). It is important to know its diagnostic possibilities compared with those of other OCT parameters, because it allows the clinicians to precise the early diagnosis, appropriate treatment and the most important for the patients—prevention of the vision loss. The

AUROC comparisons		Controls vs.			
		PPG	Early glaucoma	Moderate glaucoma	Advanced glaucoma
		p	p	p	p
Total mRNFL	Total GCL+	0.336	**0.022**	**0.024**	**0.034**
Total mRNFL	Total GCL++	0.268	0.897	0.819	1.000
Total GCL+	Total GCL++	**0.036**	**0.018**	**0.028**	**0.034**

Table 6. Comparison analysis between macular parameters' AUROC values.

results showed that this parameter also has the highest diagnostic possibilities in all perimetric glaucoma stages. These conclusions we made only after comparative analysis in diagnostic accuracy between all OCT parameters (peripapillary and macular) had been applied.

There are not many researches, which investigate macular RNFL as a separate parameter not as a part of whole ganglion cell complex. Not enough data was collected about characteristics, correlations and diagnostic possibilities of mRNFL.

In 2005 for the first time was created software algorithm for automated segmentation of retinal layers in Stratus OCT (OCT III). It helped authors differentiate four macular layers—macular nerve fiber layer (mNFL); inner retinal complex (IRC) consisting of ganglion cells, inner plexiform layer and inner nuclear layer; outer plexiform layer (OPL); outer retinal complex (ORC), consisting of outer nuclear layer, inner and outer photoreceptor segments. When the authors investigated diagnostic accuracy they found the highest values in mNFL+IRC (0.97), and lowest in OPL (0.56). Diagnostic accuracy of OPL and ORC was significantly lower from mNFL, IRC, mNFL+IRC and circumpapillary nerve fiber layer (cpNFL) ($p \leq 0.01$). They found that AUROC values of IRC, mNFL+IRC and cpNFL were significantly higher from whole retinal thickness ($p \leq 0.049$). It was not found significant differences between parameters with best diagnostic possibilities—mNFL, IRC, mNFL+IRC and cpNFL ($p \geq 0.15$). The two parameters—ORC and OPL were found also to have almost permanent thickness in patients with glaucoma in comparison with healthy volunteers [28].

In the beginning of the era "OCT diagnostics in glaucoma" was found that the whole retinal thickness decreases. Later with the initiation of spectral domain OCT (SD-OCT) in the clinical practice inner macular layers (mRNFL, GCL, IPL) were called a complex (ganglion cell complex—GCC), which consists of the bodies, dendrites and axons of the ganglion cells [29]. A self-evident fact is that GCC has significantly higher possibilities for glaucoma diagnosis than the thickness of the whole retina.

Mwanza et al. investigated diagnostic accuracy of GCIPL (ganglion cell + inner plexiform layer), RNFL ONH parameters [30]. They found that GCIPL diagnostic possibilities are between 0.918 and 0.956, and there values are comparable with the best diagnostic parameters—RNFL (between 0.933 and 0.939) and ONH parameters (0.910 and 0.962) without statistically significant difference between them.

There are two conceptions of ganglion cell loss in glaucoma. In the first—the dendrites die before the bodies, and the most resistant part of the cell of glaucoma damage are their axons. Therefore, it is reasonable to investigate the thickness of GCL + IPL separately from mRNFL. On the other hand IPL consists of the dendrites not only the ganglion cells but also the bipolar cells, and it is believed as more correctly to measure the thickness of mRNFL+GCL together.

2.5. Conclusion

Peripapillary RNFL is a proved glaucoma diagnostic parameter and also ganglion cell complex. Predominantly of the glaucoma comparisons in diagnostic accuracy are between pRNFL and GCC in different OCT devices.

The current research investigate a new SD-OCT macular parameter—mRNFL and its diagnostic possibilities for different stages of POAG. It proves that mRNFL could be used in every day clinical practice of the ophthalmologist as independent parameter with very high diagnostic possibilities for early stages of glaucoma when only structural changes are visible.

Now we are working on creating of staging system based on Total mRNFL values (cut-off values) in each glaucoma group. It could give possibilities for the ophthalmologists to use the values of this parameter in everyday clinical practice to make diagnosis and follow-up of the glaucoma patients. This grading system will be the only of the OCT structural systems created up to date. Total mRNFL has the potential to be one of the best OCT diagnostic parameters and we as researchers must find how to use it in the diagnosis of very early glaucoma changes.

Acknowledgements

We would like to acknowledge with much appreciation the crucial role of: Assoc. Prof. Todor Kundurjiev, PhD (Medical University of Sofia, Bulgaria, Department of Social Medicine and Health Management) who made the whole statistical analysis for the current research.

Conflict interest

The authors declare that there is no conflict of interest.

Notes/Thanks/Other declarations

I would like to express my special appreciation and thanks to my teacher:

Associate Professor Galina G. Dimitrova, MD, PhD.

You have been a tremendous mentor for me. I would like to thank you for encouraging my work and for allowing me to grow as a research scientist. Your advice on both science and on my clinical practice has been invaluable. I appreciate this more than you know.

Author details

Bilyana Mihaylova* and Galina Dimitrova

*Address all correspondence to: b51@abv.bg

Department of Ophthalmology, Medical University of Sofia, University Hospital 'Alexandrovska', Sofia, Bulgaria

References

[1] American Academy of Ophthalmology. Base and Clinical Science Course, 2015/2016. Section 10 - Glaucoma. Chapter 1 - Introduction to Glaucoma: Terminology, Epidemiology, and Heredity. American Academy of Ophthalmology. p16

[2] Quigley HA, Broman AT. The number of people with glaucoma worldwide in 2010 and 2020. The British Journal of Ophthalmology. 2006;**90**:262-267

[3] Quigley HA, Sanchez RM, Dunkelberger GR, et al. Chronic glaucoma selectively damages large optic nerve fibers. Investigative Ophthalmology & Visual Science. 1987;**28**(6): 913-920

[4] Tham YC, Li X, Wong TY, Quigley HA, et al. Global prevalence of glaucoma and projections of glaucoma burden through 2040: A systematic review and meta-analysis. Ophthalmology. 2014;**121**(11):2081-2090

[5] Wollstein G, Beaton S, Paunescu A, et al. Optical coherence tomography in glaucoma. In: Schuman JS, Puliafito CA, Fujimoto JG, editors. Optical Coherence Tomography of Ocular Diseases. Thorofare, NJ: SLACK Inc.; 2004. pp. 483-610

[6] Medeiros FA, Zangwill LM, Bowd C, et al. Use of progressive glaucomatous optic disk change as the reference standard for evaluation of diagnostic tests in glaucoma. American Journal of Ophthalmology. 2005;**139**:1010-1018

[7] Jonas JB, Gusek GC, Naumann GOH. Optic disk, cup and neuroretinal rim size, configuration, and correlations in normal eyes. Investigative Ophthalmology & Visual Science. 1988;**29**:1151-1158

[8] Panda-Jonas S, Jonas JB, Jakobczyk M, et al. Retinal photoreceptor count, retinal surface area, and optic disc size in normal human eyes. Ophthalmology. 1994;**101**:519-523

[9] Tanev V, Tanev IV. Possibilities for retinal nerve fiber layer visualization. In: Glaucomas. 1st ed. Steno; 2006. pp. 99-112

[10] Hood DC, Raza AS, de Moraes CG, et al. Glaucomatous damage of the macula. Progress in Retinal and Eye Research. 2013;**32**:1-21

[11] Quigley HA. Quantitative studies of retinal nerve fiber layer loss in monkey and human glaucoma. Transactions of the American Ophthalmological Society. 1987;**84**:920-966

[12] Samsonova B, Pr G-I. Analysis of factors, influencing the RNFL thickness and the optic disc rim width (Part II). Bulgarian Forum Glaucoma. 2014;**4**(5):201-207

[13] Samsonova B, Pr G-I. Analysis of factors, influencing the RNFL thickness and the optic disc rim width (Part I). Bulgarian Forum Glaucoma. 2014;**4**(4):161-168

[14] Samsonova B. Curious discrepancies between functional and structural findings in patients with glaucoma and suspicious for glaucoma (Part 1). Bulgarian Forum Glaucoma. 2013;**3**(1):10-14

[15] Samsonova B. Curious discrepancies between functional and structural findings in patients with glaucoma and suspicious for glaucoma (Part 2). Bulgarian Forum Glaucoma. 2013;**3**(2):60-72

[16] Balazsi AG, Rootman J, Drance SM, et al. The effect of age on the nerve fiber population of the human optic nerve. American Journal of Ophthalmology. 1984;**97**:760-766

[17] Mikelberg FS, Drance SM, Schuler M, et al. The normal human optic nerve. Ophthalmology. 1989;**96**:1325-1328

[18] Jonas JB, Muller-Berg JA, Schlotzer-Schrehardt UM, et al. Histomorphometry of the human optic nerve. Investigative Ophthalmology & Visual Science. 1990;**31**:736-744

[19] Jonas JB, Schmidt AM, Muller-Berg JA, et al. Human optic nerve fibre count and optic disc size. Investigative Ophthalmology & Visual Science. 1992;**33**:2012-2018

[20] Budenz DL, Anderson DR, Varma R, et al. Determinants of normal retinal nerve fiber layer thickness measured by Stratus OCT. Ophthalmology. 2007;**114**:1046-1052

[21] Xu L, Chen PP, Chen YY, et al. Quantitative nerve fiber layer measurement using scanning laser polarimetry and modulation parameters in the detection of glaucoma. Journal of Glaucoma. 1998;**7**:270-277

[22] Blumenthal EZ, Weinreb RN. Assessment of the retinal nerve fiber layer in clinical trials of glaucoma neuroprotection. Survey of Ophthalmology. 2001;**45**(Suppl 3):S305-S312; S332-S334

[23] Wu H, De Boer J, Chen T. Diagnostic capability of spectral-domain optical coherence tomography for glaucoma. American Journal of Ophthalmology. 2012;**153**(5):815-826

[24] Sommer A, Katz J, Quigley HA, et al. Clinically detectable nerve fiber atrophy precedes the onset of glaucomatous filed loss. Archives of Ophthalmology. 1991;**109**(1):77-83

[25] Harwerth RS, Carter-Dawson L, Shen F, et al. Ganglion cell losses underlying visual field defects from experimental glaucoma. Investigative Ophthalmology & Visual Science. 1999;**40**:2242-2250

[26] Hasnain SS. The missing piece in glaucoma? Open Journal of Ophthalmology. 2016;**6**: 56-62

[27] Hasnain SS. Pathogenesis of orderly loss of nerve fibers in glaucoma. Optometry: Open Access. 2016;**1**(2):110. DOI: 10.4172/2476-2075.1000110

[28] Ishikawa H, Stein DM, Wollstein G, et al. Macular segmentation with optical coherence tomography. Investigative Ophthalmology & Visual Science. 2005;**46**(6):2012-2017

[29] Tan O, Li G, Lu A, Varma R, Huang D. Advanced imaging for glaucoma study group. Mapping of macular substructures with optical coherence tomography for glaucoma diagnosis. Ophthalmology. 2008;**115**:949-956

[30] Mwanza JC, Durbin MK, Budenz DL, et al. Glaucoma diagnostic accuracy of ganglion cell–inner plexiform layer thickness: Comparison with nerve fiber layer and optic nerve head. Ophthalmology. 2012;**119**(6):1151-1158

Chapter 6

Clinical Assessment of Lesions Compressing the Visual Pathway

Lawan Abdu

Additional information is available at the end of the chapter

http://dx.doi.org/10.5772/intechopen.80277

Abstract

There is a close relationship between the visual pathway and other neuro endocrine structures. Tumours and other compressive lesions could often present with visual impairment and/or finite visual field changes. Careful clinical assessment could aid in accurate diagnosis and treatment. Pituitary gland lies in the fossa located in the sphenoid bone. Growth hormone, adreno cortico tropic hormone, and prolactin secreting adenomas could present with respective endocrine features. Optic chiasmal compression by pituitary adenoma is an indicator of suprasellar extension. Meningioma and vestigial remnant craniopharyngioma arise in the parasellar region and can compress on different parts of the optic chiasma often giving rise to classical radiological appearances and visual field changes. This includes atheroma and aneurysm of the internal carotid artery impinging on the temporal chiasma exerting direct pressure and counterpressure on the contralateral side. Others are aneurysms of the precommunicating section of the anterior cerebral artery and those of the posterior communicating artery. Compressive lesions of the visual pathway require a multi-disciplinary approach involving neurosurgeon, endocrinologist as well as the ophthalmologist.

Keywords: pituitary, adenoma, parasellar, tumours, visual, pathway

1. Introduction

The visual pathway is the anatomic channel of communication from the retinal photoreceptors where vision signals commence to their termination at the visual cortex. The photoreceptors synapse with bipolar cells (which constitute the outer nuclear layer) at the outer plexiform layer. The bipolar cells synapse with the ganglion cells at the inner plexiform layer. The ganglion cells constitute the retinal nerve fibre layer (RNFL) that enters the optic disc and collectively with the addition of apparent pupillary fibres forms the optic nerve. The ganglion nerve fibres pass through and constitute the optic nerve that has about 2.4 million afferent axons [1]. The optic nerve has an intra-ocular, intra-orbital, intra-canalicular and intra-cranial components measuring 1, 25–30, 6 and 10 mm, respectively. The optic canal entrance is about 5.5–6.5 mm and a difference of >1 mm between the two sides is unusual. The optic chiasma is about 6 mm wide and 12 mm long, it is tilted about 45° with the anterior portion being lower than posterior. In most instances (80%), the chiasma lies directly over the sella turcica. The sella is a bony cavity that houses the pituitary gland. The anterior and posterior clinoid processes bound the entrance and a piece of dura matter called the diaphragm sellae covers it. Posteriorly, the chiasma is related to the anterior part of the third ventricle (optic recess). On either side lies the extra cavernous part of the internal carotid artery. Chiasma is related above to the anterior perforating substance. Retinal nerves on reaching the optic chiasma are arranged such that fibres from the temporal half of the retina continue and join the optic tract on the same side without crossing. Inferior nasal fibres that serve superior temporal visual field cross in the anterior part of the chiasma. Such crossing fibres loop into the proximal part of the contralateral optic nerve (forming a Wilbrand's knee) before ascending the optic tract. The superior nasal fibres (that sub-serve the inferior nasal field of vision) cross the chiasma posteriorly before ascending the contralateral optic tract. Macular fibres cross throughout the chiasma. Crossed nerve fibres terminate at layers 1, 4, 6 of the lateral geniculate body while uncross fibres terminate at layers 2, 3, 5. From the lateral geniculate body arise the geniculocalcarine nerve fibres that form the optic radiations that terminate in the visual cortex. As the fibres proceed more posteriorly, those from corresponding retinal points are brought close together thus ensuring binocular single vision and stereopsis.

2. Intra-orbital and intra-canalicular optic nerve compression

The optic nerve can be compressed in the intra-orbital portion by inflammatory conditions of the orbit such as idiopathic inflammatory pseudo-tumour and thyroid-related orbitopathy (TRO). TRO is associated with increased orbital volume from extra-ocular muscle enlargement particularly the medial rectus and such occurrence is predictive of compressive dysthyroid optic neuropathy (DON) [2]. DON could precede, occur simultaneously or even after control of symptoms of hyperthyroidism. In the presence of toxic hyperthyroidism, the ocular signs such as lid lag/retraction, proptosis and the typical open staring facies are present in addition to the systemic features. Increased orbital volume leads to restrictive myopathy and pupillary dilation unresponsive to light stimulation is a pointer to optic nerve damage with eventual optic atrophy. This can present with marked reduction in vision even in the absence of exposure keratopathy. After clinical and hormonal evaluation, treatment involves graded and tapered doses of steroids and orbital decompression. Rapamycin, a fibroblast and T cell inhibitor, has been shown to be effective in improving visual acuity, colour plate test and visual fields when dysthyroid orbital inflammation is refractory to steroid and orbital decompression [3].

Intra-canalicular optic nerve may be compressed by optic nerve glioma, meningioma or schwannoma. Although quite rare, isolated optic nerve glioma poses a special challenge in ensuring vision preservation at the same time achieving tumour control [4]. The tumour could present in child or adulthood with progressive painless vision loss and axial proptosis.

http://dx.doi.org/10.5772/intechopen.80277

There could be a demonstrable apparent pupillary defect and a scotoma on the affected side. The contralateral eye may be normal. Children with sporadic optic pathway glioma have a poorer visual prognosis than those with neurofibromatosis (NF-1) [5]. Diagnosis is based on clinical neuroradiological assessment. Serial scanning is required to detect changes in size and or extent. Chemotherapy is an option to be considered. Pattern visual evoked potential (VEP) and pattern electroretinograms (ERGs) provide early objective indication of optic nerve dysfunction even in the presence of unchanged neuroradiological features [6]. **Figure 1** is a CT scan coronal section of right optic nerve glioma.

2.1. Compression of the optic chiasma by pituitary tumours

The pituitary gland lies in the pituitary fossa, a bony cavity in the sphenoid bone. In most instances, the optic chiasma is positioned directly above the sella turcica. The pituitary gland has an anterior and a posterior portion. The anterior portion has a variety of cells that secrete different hormones. The acidophil cells produce growth hormone (GH), basophil cells produce adrenocorticotropic hormone (ACTH), while the chromophobe "C"-cells produce prolactin. Tumours secreting luteinizing hormone (LH) and thyroid stimulating hormones (TSH) are extremely rare to deserve a mention. Pituitary tumours have both endocrine and ophthalmological manifestations. Pituitary adenomas represent 15% of primary brain tumours and visual disturbances arising from local mass effect on the visual system are common clinical manifestation [7]. In some instances, more so with younger patients, vision lost is more frequent (39%) followed by endocrine abnormality (21%), and headache (15%). Bitemporal visual field defects were the most prevalent (41%) [8]. Common neuro-ophthalmic manifestations include blurred vision, impairment in colour vision, relative afferent pupillary defect, optic atrophy headache and bitemporal field defect [9]. A study showed that the size of the pituitary adenoma has bearing on its effect as those larger than 2 cm cause defects in vision while those 2 cm or smaller do not cause significant visual impairment [10].

A growth hormone secreting adenoma manifesting before closure of the epiphyseal plate is characterised by gigantism and after puberty it causes acromegaly. Such patients often notice

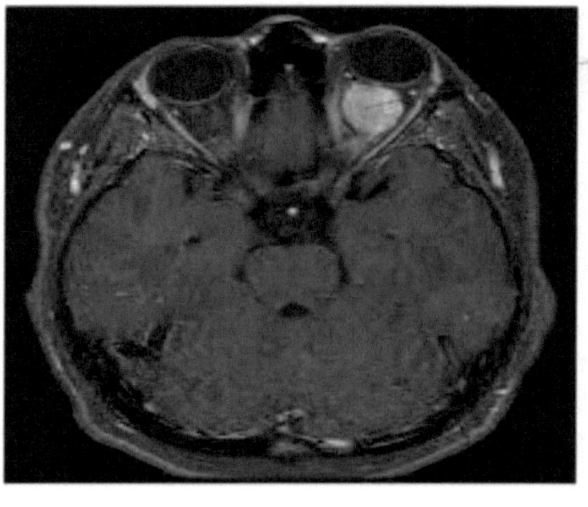

Figure 1. Coronal CT scan showing optic nerve glioma.

their shoe, hat, clothes and ring do not fit. Other features include skin (hyperhidrosis and hirsutism in females), hoarseness of the voice and malocclusion due to jaw enlargement. The clinical features are quite obvious in most instances.

ACTH secreting basophil adenoma is characterised by fat mal-distribution giving rise to hump back and swollen "moon-shaped" face. Other features include skin striations and sign of fluid retention, easy bruising and slow wound healing. In the presence of elevated serum cortisol, the entity is described as Cushing's syndrome. Such patients are prone to developing diabetes mellitus, hypertension and osteoporosis. A paradoxical rise in GH level is observed in response to oral glucose tolerance test in contrast to normal individuals in whom there is suppression of the hormone to below 2 mU/L.

Chromophobe adenomas are the most common primary intra-cranial tumours and when prolactin secreting is named prolactinoma, the tumour present in early adulthood or middle age. The tumour causes infertility, amenorrhea and galactorrhea in females. Males could present with loss of libido, impotence, infertility and breast signs similar to females.

2.2. Craniopharyngioma

Craniopharyngioma arises from the vestigial remnants of Rathke's pouch along the path of the pituitary stalk. The tumour present in children with delayed sexual development and dwarfism, and in adults, visual impairment and field defects are common. Craniopharyngioma often causes visual loss due to the tumour's close relation to the anterior visual pathways [11]. The tumour compresses the chiasma from above and behind affecting the superior nasal fibres and giving rise to bitemporal hemianopia dense inferiorly and progresses clockwise in the left eye and anticlockwise in the right eye. The tumour gives raise to supra sella calcification and may have cystic areas.

In general, some hormone-secreting pituitary tumours may present with endocrine features in the early stages before headache and signs of chiasmal compression manifest. Patient may present with visual impairment which could be progressive in nature. As the tumour expands, it reaches the diaphragma sellae. The dura structure has pain sensing fibres and stretching results in non-specific headache. With further growth, the tumour breaks through the diaphragma and the headache stops. Presence of headache indicates supra sella extension of pituitary tumour. Pituitary tumours compress the chiasma at its anterior portion. Therefore, the inferior nasal fibres are affected first and subsequently the superior nasal fibres. Visual filed assessment would reveal a bitemporal hemianopia dense superiorly and progressing anticlockwise in the left eye and clockwise in the right eye as shown in **Figure 2**. Diagnosis is aided by clinical evaluation, perimetry, hormonal assay and radiological investigations.

MRI is the radiological investigation of choice although in resource-scarce sub-Saharan Africa, it is not accessible to most clinicians. Therefore, digital X-ray and CT scan are more readily available and affordable. MRI demonstrates presence of a mass lesion and its relation to the optic chiasma. Coronal section demonstrates contents of the sella turcica, while sagittal sections can be obtained through the chiasma and optic nerve (before and after gadolinium injection which is known to enhance pituitary adenomas), and axial scans. Radiological features with the presence of identifiable and quantifiable space occupying mass which may erode the sellae floor or clinoid

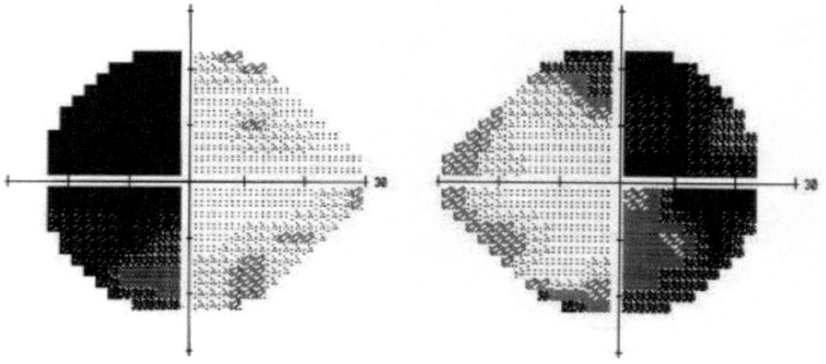

Figure 2. Bitemporal hemianopia dense superiorly.

processes cause widening of the inter clinoid space and may cause supra sellae calcification. Calcification in pituitary adenoma is rare (a report indicates occurrence in 5.6%); therefore, preoperative radiological calcification should not be a decider regarding surgical intervention [11].

On MRI, craniopharyngioma shows an isodense lesion on T1 images, while cystic components appear hyperintense. It also causes oedema that spread along the optic tracts [12]. For most of the tumours irrespective of the imaging technique use to evaluate the patient, there is a direct link between visual defect and chiasmal compression [13].

2.3. Meningioma

Meningioma that accounts for one-third of primary intracranial tumours [14] typically affects middle-aged women and could arise at the tuberculum, the sphenoid ridge or olfactory groove. Sphenoidal ridge meningioma compresses the optic nerve early if positioned medially. When present in the sphenoid bone and mid-cranial fossa, the vision is affected later and patient may have temporal fullness as a result of reactive hyperostosis.

Tuberculum meningioma (**Figure 3**) compresses proximal part of the ipsilateral optic nerve giving rise to ipsilateral scotoma and a crescent-shaped junctional scotoma in the contra lateral eye due to its effect on the looped crossed inferior nasal fibres (Wilbrand's knee) as illustrated in **Figure 4**. Olfactory groove meningioma affects both vision and sense of smell. CT scan may show new bone formation due to reactive hyperostosis.

2.4. Treatment of pituitary and other parasellar tumours

The type, size, site, nature, presentation and associated clinical complexity of the tumour determine the best modality of treatment. Treatment of growth hormone secreting adenoma is necessary due to associated mortality from metabolic [15], circulatory impairments and cancer [16] apart from visual pathway compression. IGF-1 lowering medications can be used although surgical options like trans-sphenoidal trans-cranial surgery have been in practice. Stereotactic radio surgery (SRS) has been found to be a definitive treatment option for patients with persistent or recurrent acromegaly after surgical resection [17].

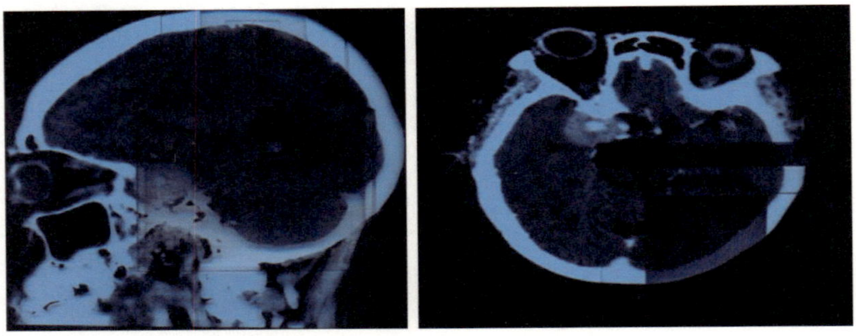

Figure 3. CT scan showing tuberculum sellae meningioma with areas of hyperostosis.

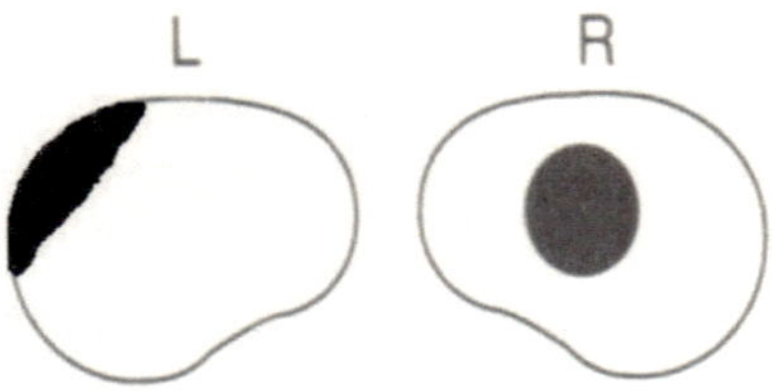

Figure 4. Ipsilateral scotoma with contralateral junctional scotoma.

ACTH secreting pituitary adenoma is amenable to trans-sphenoidal surgery as the first line of treatment. Some patients may not achieve cure, while others have recurrence warranting use of medication such as the recently approved pasireotide, a somatostatin receptor ligand [18].

Traditionally, prolactin-secreting pituitary adenoma is treated with bromocriptine, a dopamine agonist, though the drug has been implicated in predisposing the patient to pituitary apoplexy. This complication is less with cabergoline therapy. Trans-sphenoidal surgery can be performed to relieve visual impairment [19].

Gross total resection of craniopharyngioma is the aim of treatment [20]; failure of which requires adjunct radiotherapy. Intra-cavity radiotherapy using phosphorus-32 (^{32}P) colloid has been tried in cystic craniopharyngioma [21]. There is a reported case of vision recovery after endoscopic transplanum transtuberculum resection of a craniopharyngioma [22].

Meningioma can be an asymptomatic benign disease. Tumour growth is experienced in two-thirds of patients and a third may eventually require neurosurgical interventions. Gamma knife surgery (GKS) can control the tumour clinically and radiologically [23]. Radiotherapy remains one of the most relevant therapeutic options for the treatment patients with meningioma [14].

2.5. Vascular chiasmal compression

The internal carotid artery (ICA) on emerging from the cavernous sinus ascends upwards in close relation to the underneath of the proximal part of the optic nerve. ICA curves posteriorly and upwards on the lateral edge of the optic chiasma. The pre-communicating branch of the

http://dx.doi.org/10.5772/intechopen.80277

anterior cerebral artery crosses the chiasma close to its junction with the optic nerve. The posterior communicating artery passes backwards under the optic tract to join the posterior cerebral artery. An atheroma of the internal carotid artery can compress the chiasma laterally and also impinge it on the contralateral giving rise to binasal hemianopia and the defect is not often symmetrical as illustrated in **Figure 5**. Aneurysm of the ICA, pre-communicating segment of the anterior cerebral and posterior cerebral arteries, could give rise to binasal hemianopia [24].

2.6. Visual field defects in retrochiasmal pathway lesions

2.6.1. Optic tract

Brain tumours and aneurysm can affect the retrochiasmal visual pathway giving rise to varied visual field defects [25, 26]. The optic tract arises from the posterior aspect of the chiasma and extends posteriorly around the cerebral peduncle to reach the lateral geniculate body (LGB). It consists of crossed nasal fibres and ipsilateral temporal fibres. Compression results in bilateral hemifield loss opposite to the side of the lesion. The homonymous hemianopia may be complete or incomplete but incongruous as nerve fibres from corresponding retinal points are not closely related. Compression of the LGB similarly results in asymmetrical hemianopic visual field defect. The optic tract contains both visual and pupillomotor fibres. The visual fibres terminate at the LGB, while pupillary fibres leave the tract anterior to the LGB pass through the brachium to reach the pretectal nucleus at the level of the superior colliculus. Tract lesion can give rise to afferent pupillary defect, thus the pupil contracts when the unaffected side of the retina is stimulated with light, but not so when the affected hemiretina is stimulated (Wernicke's hemianopic pupil). In clinical practice, this is difficult to demonstrate due to scattering of light shone on the retina unless a pinpoint source of light is used. The ganglion cells from the retina terminate at the LGB; therefore, tract lesion can result in optic atrophy. In this instance, the ipsilateral disc manifests atrophy of the superior and inferior aspects (due to effect on temporal fibres), while the contralateral disc shows atrophy of the nasal and temporal neuroretinal rim "bow tie atrophy" due to effect on the nasal retinal fibres. Typical homonymous hemianopic field loss is shown in **Figure 6**.

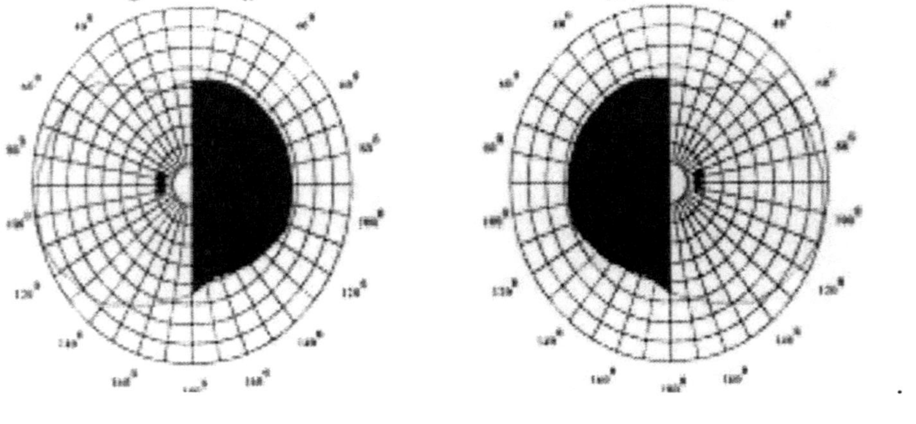

Figure 5. Binasal hemianopia in vascular chiasmal compression.

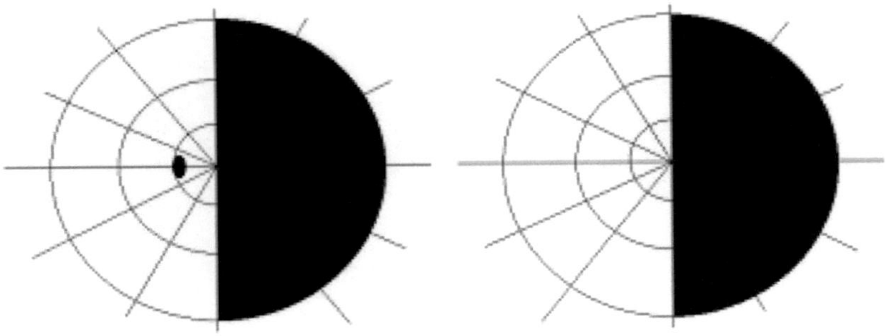

Figure 6. Homonymous hemianopia.

2.6.2. *Optic radiations*

The geniculocalcarine fibres arise from the LGB to the striate cortex located on the medal aspect of the occipital cortex above and below the calcarine fissure. As the fibres spread posteriorly, nerves from corresponding retinal points are brought close together so that incomplete hemianopia caused by lesions in the posterior radiations is more congruous than those located anteriorly. The middle and posterior cerebral arteries provide dual blood supply to the optic radiations and visual cortex.

2.6.3. *Main radiations*

The main radiations are related to the occipital horn of the lateral ventricle and the trigone. Compression at this location results in complete homonymous hemianopia. Optokinetic nystagmus (OKN) involves smooth pursuit movement followed by a saccade in the opposite direction of the initial movement as the eye fixate on the next target. In homonymous hemianopia, due to parietal lobe lesions, the smooth pursuit movement towards side of the lesion is defective.

2.6.4. *Temporal radiations*

The visual defects observed in lesion of the temporal radiations are homonymous superior quadrantanopia (described as "pie in the sky") illustrated in **Figure 7**. There may be associated

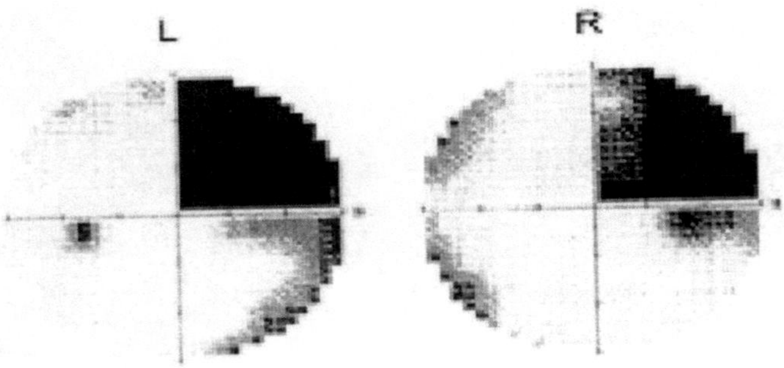

Figure 7. Superior quadrantanopia—"pie in the sky".

hemiparesis and sensory loss on the affected side due to close relation of the radiations with sensory-motor fibres of the internal capsule.

2.6.5. *Anterior parietal radiations*

The superior nasal fibres that sub-serve the inferior temporal visual fields pass through the parietal lobe; therefore, lesions of the anterior parietal radiations result in contralateral congruous homonymous inferior quadrantanopia (described as "pie on the floor") as shown in **Figure 8**.

2.6.6. *Striate cortex*

Peripheral visual fields are represented anteriorly (supplied by posterior cerebral artery), while central macula vision is posteriorly located lateral to the tip of the calcarine cortex and supplied by a branch of the middle cerebral artery. Anteriorly located lesions of the striate cortex will result in congruous homonymous hemianopia. If the cause has a vascular component, the macular vision is spared as shown in **Figure 9**.

Figure 10 shows congruous macular homonymous hemianopia typical of lesions of the tip of the occipital cortex.

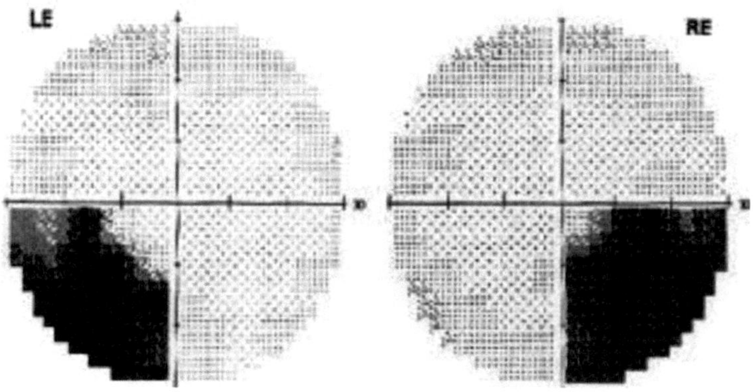

Figure 8. Inferior quadrantanopia—"pie on the floor".

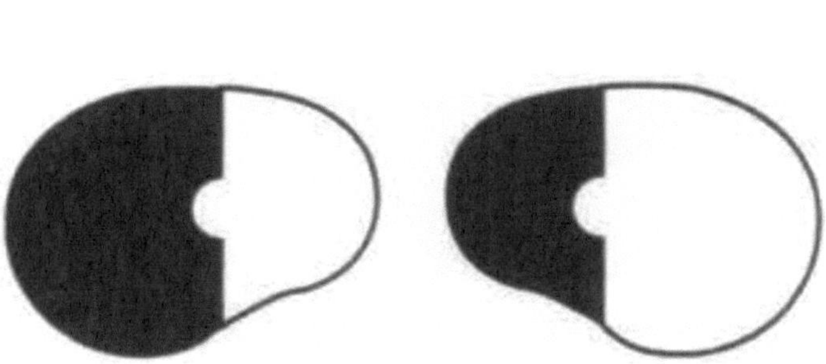

Figure 9. Congruous homonymous hemianopia with macular sparing.

2.6.7. Conclusion

Compressive lesions affecting the visual pathway could present with variety of visual impairments. Hormone-secreting adenoma can present with endocrine features in addition to visual field changes. **Figure 11** is an illustration of some of different causes and the associated visual fields.

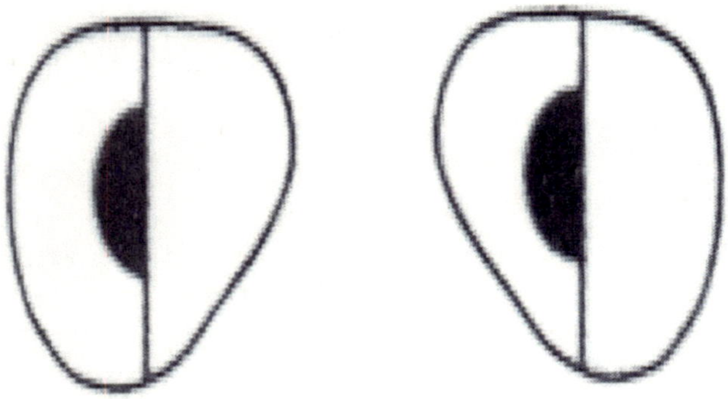

Figure 10. Congruous macular homonymous hemianopia.

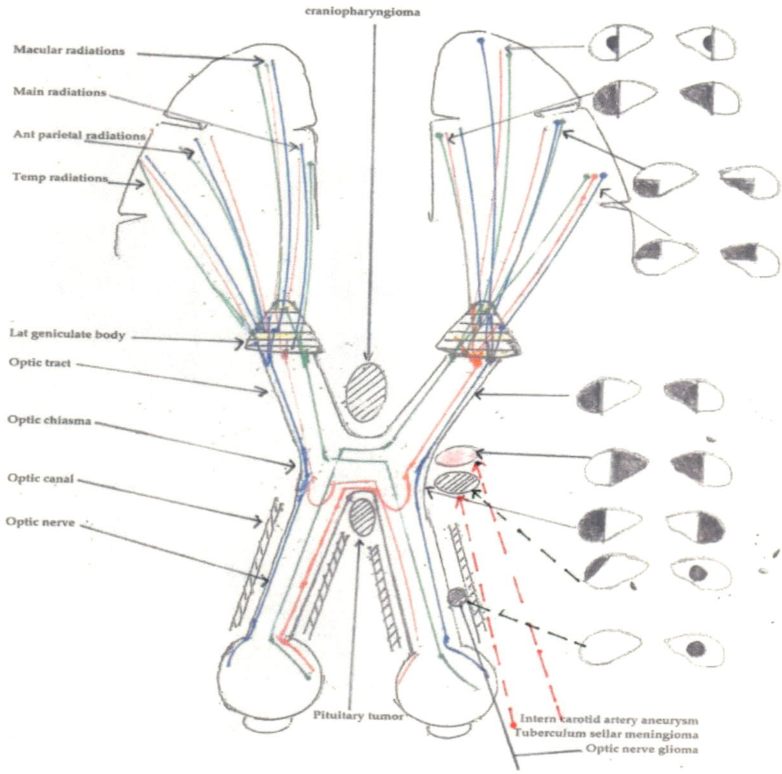

Figure 11. A diagram of the visual pathway showing location of some of the lesions and the associated field changes.

http://dx.doi.org/10.5772/intechopen.80277

Acknowledgements

Appreciation to my employer Bayero University Kano—Nigeria for creating an enabling academic environment.

Conflict of interest

None.

Author details

Lawan Abdu

Address all correspondence to: lawal1966@yahoo.com

Department of Ophthalmology, Faculty of Clinical Sciences, College of Health Sciences, Bayero University Kano, Nigeria

References

[1] Jost BJ, Andreas MS, Jens AM, et al. Human optic nerve fiber count and optic disc size. Investigative Ophthalmology & Visual Science. 1992;**32**(6):2012-2018

[2] Weis E, Heran MK, Jhamb A, et al. Quantitative computed tomographic predictors of compressive optic neuropathy in patients with thyroid orbitopathy: A volumetric analysis. Ophthalmology. 2012;**119**(10):2174-2178

[3] Chang S, Perry JD, Kosmorsky GS, et al. Rapamycin for treatment of refractory dysthyroid compressive optic neuropathy. Ophthalmic Plastic & Reconstructive Surgery. 2007;**23**(3):225-226

[4] Hamideh D, Hoehn ME, Harreld JH, et al. Isolated optic nerve glioma in children with and without neurofibromatosis: Retrospective characterization and analysis of outcomes. Journal of Child Neurology. 2018;**33**(6):375-382

[5] Glaser JS. Topical diagnosis: The optic chiasma. In: Glaser JS, editor. Neuro-Ophthalmology. Philadelphia: Lippincott Williams & Wilkins; 1999. p. 99

[6] Moradi P, Robson AG, Rose GE, et al. Electrophysiological monitoring in a patient with an optic nerve glioma. Documenta Ophthalmologica. 2008;**117**(2):171-174

[7] Fredes F, Undurraga G, Rojas P, et al. Visual outcomes after endoscopic pituitary surgery in patients presenting with preoperative visual deficits. Journal of Neurological Surgery. Part B, Skull Base. 2017;**78**(6):461-465

[8] Ogra S, Nichols AD, Stylli S, et al. Visual acuity and pattern of visual field loss at presentation in pituitary adenoma. Journal of Clinical Neuroscience. 2014;**21**(5):735-740

[9] Tagoe NN, Essuman VA, Fordjuor G, et al. Neuro-ophthalmic and clinical characteristics of brain tumours in a tertiary Hospital in Ghana. Ghana Medical Journal. 2015;**49**(3): 181-186

[10] Ho RW, Huang HM, Ho JT. The influence of pituitary adenoma size on vision and visual outcomes after trans-sphenoidal adenectomy: A report of 78 cases. Journal of Korean Neurosurgical Association. 2015;**57**(1):23-31

[11] Ogiwara T, Nagm A, Yamamoto Y, et al. Clinical characteristics of pituitary adenomas with radiological calcification. Acta Neurochirurgica. 2017;**159**(11):2187-2192

[12] Nagahata M, Hosoya T, Kayama T, et al. Edema along the optic tract: A useful MR finding for the diagnosis of craniopharyngiomas. AJNR. American Journal of Neuroradiology. 1998;**19**(9):1753-1757

[13] Huang WC, Lee LS. Visual field defects in patients with pituitary adenomas. Zhonghua Yi Xue Za Zhi (Taipei). 1997;**60**(5):245-251

[14] Pinzi V, Bisogno I, Prada F, et al. Radiotherapy of meningioma: A treatment in need of radiobiological research. International Journal of Radiation Biology. 2018;**18**:1-23

[15] Ku CR, Choe EY, Hong JW, et al. No differences in metabolic outcomes between nadir GH 0.4 and 1.0 ng/mL during OGTT in surgically cured acromegalic patients (Observational study). Medicine (Baltimore). 2016;**95**(24):e3808

[16] Esposito D, Ragnarsson O, Granfeldt D, et al. Decreasing mortality and changes in treatment patterns in patients with acromegaly from a nationwide study. European Journal of Endocrinology. 2018;**178**(5):459-469

[17] Ding D, Mehta GU, Patibandla MR, et al. Stereotactic radiosurgery for acromegaly: An international multicenter retrospective cohort study. Neurosurgery 2018 May 10. DOI: 10.1093/neuros/nyy178. [Epub ahead of print]

[18] Langlois F, Chu J, Fleseriu M. Pituitary-directed therapies for Cushing's disease. Frontiers in Endocrinology (Lausanne). 2018;**1**(9):164. DOI: 10.3389/fendo.2018.00164. eCollection 2018

[19] Ghadirian H, Shirani M, Ghazi-Mirsaeed S, et al. Pituitary apoplexy during treatment of prolactinoma with cabergoline. Asian Journal of Neurosurgery. 2018;**13**(1):93-95

[20] Guo F, Wang G, Suresh V, et al. Clinical study on microsurgical treatment for craniopharyngioma in a single institutional series of 335 patients. Clinical Neurology and Neurosurgery. 2018;**167**:162-172

[21] Chang H, Zhang J, Cao W, et al. Drug distribution and clinical safety in treating cystic craniopharyngiomas using intracavitary radiotherapy with phosphorus-32 colloid. Oncology Letters. 2018;**15**(4):4997-5003

[22] Todeschini AB, Montaser AS, Shahein M, et al. Endoscopic endonasal approach to a suprasellar craniopharyngioma. Journal of Neurological Surgery. Part B, Skull Base. 2018;**79**(Suppl 3):S237-S238

[23] Kim KH, Kang SJ, Choi JW, et al. Clinical and radiological outcomes of proactive gamma knife surgery for asymptomatic meningiomas compared with the natural course without intervention. Journal of Neurosurgery. 2018;**18**:1-10

[24] O'Connell JEA, Du Boulay EDGH. Binasal hemianopia. Journal of Neurology, Neurosurgery, and Psychiatry. 1973;**36**(5):697-709

[25] Rico G, Smith SV, Siddiqui Y, Whyte A, et al. Neuro-ophthalmologic manifestations of cholangiocarcinoma: A case series. Eye (London, England). 2017;**31**(8):1245-1248

[26] Zorić Geber M, Krolo I, Zrinscak O, et al. Unruptured giant intracranial aneurysm of the internal carotid artery: Late ocular symptoms. Seminars in Ophthalmology. 2016;**31**(3):291-294

Chapter 7

Contribution to the Optic Nerve

Marija Radenković

Additional information is available at the end of the chapter

http://dx.doi.org/10.5772/intechopen.80278

Abstract

Optic nerve head drusen (ONHD) represent congenital anomaly, which is a form of calcium degeneration of optic nerve head axons. They are initially asymptomatic but may causes progressive optic neuropathy. They are presented as acellular, hyaline deposits of globular appearance in front of the lamina cribrosa (prelaminar segment). They are formed due to altered axonal transport, small diameter of scleral canal, direct compression, or ischemia. Frequent complications: progressive visual field scotoma, ischemic optic neuropathy, central retinal artery or vein occlusion, and neovascularization adjacent to the optic nerve head. Useful diagnostic tools ophthalmoscopy, angiography, standard automated perimetry, B-scan ultrasonography, CT, OCT, HRT, GDx, and electrophysiological examination. Therapeutic procedures are medical, laser, and surgical. Pilot studies confirmed benefit of topical hypotensive drugs even when drusen are not associated with glaucoma. By reducing intraocular pressure, the compression to the optic nerve axons decreases, thus improving perfusion of the optic nerve head. The paper presents young female patient with bilateral optic nerve drusen and progressive visual field defects (scotomas), which implies topical hypotensive therapy. After 6 months scotoma and loss of sensitivity of the visual field were reduced. Neuroprotective drugs are investigated to reduce potential visual morbidity.

Keywords: optic nerve head, drusen, visual field, topical hypotensive drug, glaucoma

1. Introduction

Optic nerve head drusen (ONHD) represent the congenital, developmental anomaly of the second cranial nerve. This is a form of calcium degeneration of the axons of the optic nerve head (ONH). They are initially asymptomatic, but are not so rare and can cause lower visual acuity. Thus, they are also considered to be one of the causes of the progressive type of optic neuropathy with genetic etiology [1, 2].

Their occurrence is most common in 3.4–37 per 1000 adult white people (0.34–3.7%), with a frequent bilateral presentation in 75–85% of all cases [3, 4]. They are less common in black people, equally represented among the sexes, while the average prevalence in the pediatric population is 0.4% [5–7].

For the first time, they were histologically recognized by Heinrich Muller in the nineteenth century (1858) [8, 9]. Clinically, they were described with the contribution of Liebreich in 1868, only 17 years after the construction of the direct ophthalmoscope [10]. A detailed structure was described by Tso in 1967. The author also postulates the pathophysiological mechanisms of the formation and evolution of the drusen [11].

Genetically, optic nerve head drusen are inherited in autosomal dominant (AD) type of inheritance with variable penetration. Lorentzen et al. founded that the incidence of drusen is 10 times higher among members of the family with manifest optic nerve drusen [9]. Drusen may occur primarily isolated or associated with the eye (angioid streaks, retinitis pigmentosa, open-angle glaucoma, etc.) (**Table 1**) or as systemic diseases (pseudoxanthoma elasticum (PXE) or Gronblad-Strandberg syndrome, Usher syndrome, Noonan syndrome, etc.) (**Table 2**) [7, 12]. Antclif et al. state that the inheritance of a small diameter (disk area) of the optic nerve head is a risk factor for formation of optic nerve head drusen. The small optic disk (ONH) and mesodermal dysplasia result in vascular dysplasia and therefore are considered as significant causative factors. Optic disk drusen are more commonly present in vascular and/or structural developmental anomalies of the ONH. Among the vascular anomalies, the most frequent patterns of disorders are two and three branches of blood vessels, cilioretinal artery, and optociliary shunt [9, 11].

Acquired myelinated nerve fibers
Aneurysm of the ophthalmic artery
Astrocytic hamartoma
Best's vitelliform macular dystrophy
β-thalassemia
Birdshot chorioretinopathy
Combined hamartoma of the retina and retinal pigment epithelium
Congenital night blindness
Familial macular dystrophy
Glaucoma
Gyrate atrophy
Idiopathic intracranial hypertension
Idiopathic parafoveal telangiectasia
Morning glory disk anomaly
Ocular tumoral calcinosis

Optic nerve tumors
Peripapillary central serous retinopathy
Pigmented paravenous retinochoroidal atrophy (PPRCA)
Pseudoxanthoma elasticum and angioid streaks
Retinitis pigmentosa
Severe early childhood onset retinal dystrophy (SECORD)
Tilted optic disk
Tubulointerstitial nephritis and uveitis (TINU) syndrome

Table 1. Ocular diseases associated with optic nerve head drusen.

Alport syndrome
Cystic fibrosis
Delayed language development and dyslexia
Down syndrome
Headache and seizure disorders
Psychomotor retardation
Schizophrenia
Sturge-Weber syndrome
Teeth and jaw anomalies
Trisomy 15q
Tuberous sclerosis

Table 2. Systemic diseases associated with optic nerve head drusen.

Optic nerve head drusen are acellular, hyaline deposits of globular appearance in the prelaminar segment of the optic nerve head, usually below the level of the Bruch membrane of the surrounding retina. They are formed of amino and nucleic acids, mucopolysaccharides, calcium, and iron. They represent a dynamic structure, which increases during lifetime due to calcium deposition and consequent compression of the surrounding axons [4, 11]. Among the etiological factors for optic nerve drusen formation are altered axonal transport, the small diameter of the scleral canal and the ONH, direct compression, and ischemia [4, 13].

Tso states that altered axonal metabolism causes intracellular calcification of the mitochondria, degeneration and rupture of the axons with extrusion, and deposition of mitochondrial content into the extracellular space. Seitz points out that slow antero- and/or retrograde axoplasmic transport initiates the disintegration of the axons with subsequent calcium deposition and accumulation. The small diameter of the scleral canal and the specific anatomy of the

ONH compromise the axoplasmic transport. Mechanical compression causes delay of axonal transport (stasis) [5, 11, 14]. In the younger age, optic nerve drusen are near to the lamina cribrosa, and they are overlapped by nerve and vascular structures and are called *hidden* (*buried*). Optic nerve head drusen during life, become visible, and are elevated in predilected nasal-lower sector of the ONH.

Clinical classification of ONH drusen is as follows:

Grade I: deep, hidden formations

Grade II: visible separated drusen (1–6)

Grade III: dense prominent drusen (> 6) with an unclear border ONH [4, 15]

Most patients are asymptomatic for a long time. Rarely, they can have transient visual obscurations in the form of a flicker (9%) but often are associated with progressive visual field defects (scotoma) and relative afferent pupillary defect (RAPD) in advanced cases. The incidence of visual field defects in adults with drusen is 24–87%. Visual field scotoma can be an arcuate, peripheral enlargement of the blind spot, a less frequent nasal step, and a constriction of the visual field. The central visual acuity is preserved for a long time; although after a long lasting of narrowed visual field, sudden loss of central vision is possible, thus indicating complications [11, 16, 17].

Besides visual field defects due to the compression of the retinal ganglion cells' axons, numerous vascular complications due to ischemia may occur, such as non-arteritic ischemic optic neuropathy (NAION); central retinal artery occlusion (CRAO); branch or central retinal vein occlusion (BRVO, CRVO); intravitreal, subretinal, and flamed disk hemorrhage; maculopathy; and neovascularization adjacent to the optic nerve head [4, 16, 18].

The diagnosis is made by clinical examination and additional investigation. Superficial drusen are yellowish-oval prominent structures that give an unclear appearance of the ONH border, and they are considered as the main cause of pseudoedema. Additional methods, photofundus and fluorescein angiography, fundus autofluorescence, computerized perimetry (SAP), B-scan ultrasonography, OCT (EDI-OCT, SS-OCT, OCT angiography), HRT, GDx, computerized tomography (CT), and electrophysiological testing, are applied in the confirmation of hidden or superficial drusen [7, 16, 18].

Differential diagnosis is significant if pseudoedema of ONH drusen is suspected in aim to distinct numerous causes of the true edema of ONH: inflammatory, stagnant, or ischemic etiology. Buried drusen frequently produce elevation of the optic nerve head and obscuration of the margins, making it difficult to distinguish buried drusen from true papilledema based solely on funduscopic examination. However, during examination, it could be noticed that in true papilledema, the optic nerve head swelling extends into the peripapillary retina, causing RNFL thickening and consequently obscuration of the peripapillary vasculature. In contrast, elevation from optic nerve head drusen is confined to the optic nerve disk. In the case of pseudoedema, the absence of optic nerve head hyperemia, obscuration of surface arteries, exudates, venous congestion, cotton-wool spots, and peripapillary circumferential subretinal fluid lines (Patton's lines) may help distinguish optic nerve head drusen from true papilledema [7, 19].

In differential diagnosis angiography could be helpful equally. While profuse leakage is apparent in the early angiographic phases of the edematous optic nerve head, the drusen optic nerve should never leak. However, there is late staining of the nerve on the angiogram. It is important not to mistake this late staining for leakage in the early phase; besides an autofluorescence phenomenon and OCT ONH features can help to secure this diagnosis [20].

Therapy can be medical, laser, and surgical. There is no generally accepted and approved therapeutic protocol that is applied in the case of the ONH. Monitoring is advised in asymptomatic patients, while the application of any therapeutic modality is determined by potential complications of the drusen. A large number of studies confirm the benefit of topical hypotensive drugs even in cases where ONH drusen are not associated with glaucoma. With the reduction of intraocular pressure is achieved, which reduces mechanical pressure on the axons of the optic nerve, indirectly the reperfusion as main goal is acheived. Choroidal neovascular membranes (CNV) adjacent to the optic nerve are treated with anti-VEGF or laser therapy [12, 16, 21]. The proposed surgical therapeutic modality, radial optic neurotomia, was used to decompress the head of the optic nerve due to ischemic neuropathy. The method was described by Opremcak (2001) in the treatment of CRVO and was also applied to progressive scotoma caused by drusen. Also successful and unsuccessful excision of drusen was reported but rarely applied [21–25].

The main aim is to provide recent data of etiology, epidemiology, pathology, diagnosis, and potential treatment of optic nerve head drusen. All relevant data was collected by investigation in small samples or individual cases and reports. There is no major controlled clinical trial on therapeutic effects and protocol in drusen, but there are numerous individual reports of topical hypotensive drug benefit. The author presents the case from personal clinical praxis and the effect of hypotensive drug. The presentation is followed with the discussion of current knowledge and recommendations that are based on individual evaluation. The largest investigation found was in Grippo's study on 60 patients (13 hypertensive and 47 normotensive eyes). Therefore this is not a general therapeutic protocol, just individually based potential recommendation.

2. Case presentation

A young female (20 years old), without prior ophthalmological or systemic disease, was referred to the ophthalmologist at the eye clinic due to changes in optic nerve of her left eye. Clinical examination showed normal visual acuity (Snellen chart) and anterior segment:

VOD = cc −2.0 DSph = 1.0; VOS = cc −2.50 DSph = 0.9–1.0; and TOU = 14–18 mmHg.

CCT OU = 616 μm (−5 mmHg factor for correction).

Indirect ophthalmoscopy of the left eye showed unclear ONH borders, globular appearance, more prominent nasally (**Figure 1**).

In further observation, we performed echosonography (ultrasound A/B scanner UD-6000, Tomey) and B-scan OU: oval ONH changes of high reflectivity. FAG: the time of the arm-retina was regular. Blood vessels are completely and on time filled with contrast. Diffuse, oval, partially confluent changes with autofluorescence of the optic nerve head in the left eye (**Figures 2** and **3**).

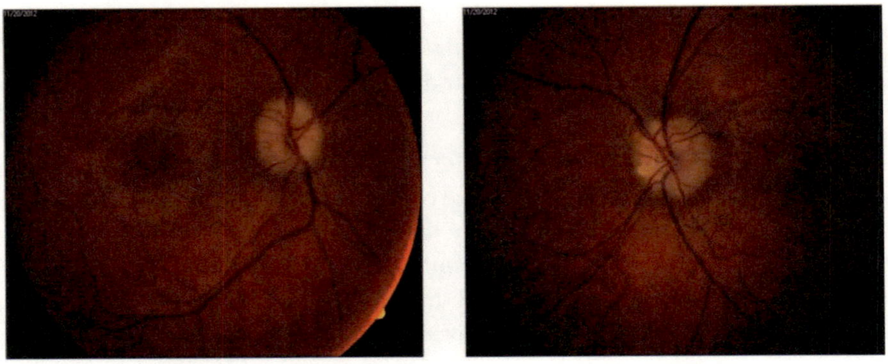

(A) (B)

Figure 1. Photofundus OD (A) and OS (B): an unclear ONH border with superficial drusen.

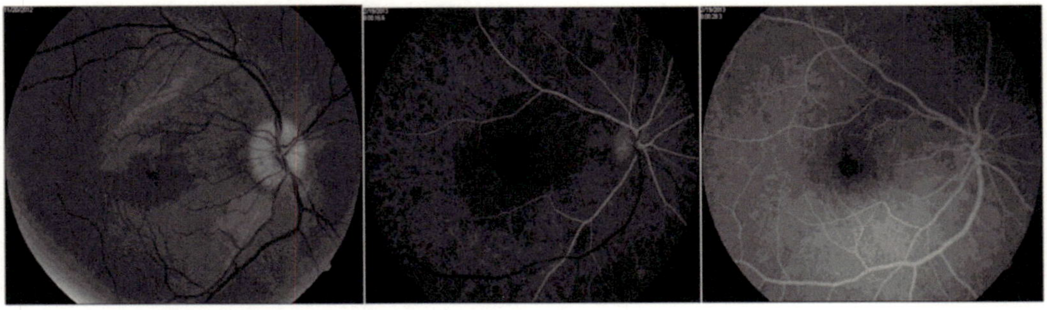

Figure 2. FAG OD: finding normal.

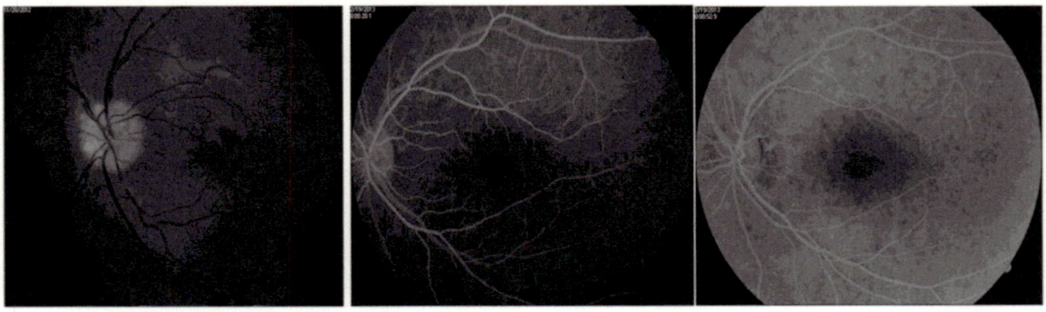

Figure 3. FAG OS: confluent autofluorescent ONH changes.

A standard automatic perimetry (Humphrey visual field analyzer, threshold test 30-2; 24-2) was performed, and scotoma progression in the visual field of both eyes was observed in four successive testing over 1 year. The most frequent defect is confluent, relative, and absolute paracentral scotoma, up to the central 15° (in the right eye; constriction of visual field) and inferior nasal quadrantanopia (left eye). After that finding, topical hypotensive therapy (brimonidine 0.2%, which was replaced by latanoprost 0.005% after 3 months due to allergic reaction) was applied (**Figures 4–7**).

HRT detects marginal thinning in the nasal sector of the left eye (**Figure 8**).

RNFL examination OCT (Stratus optical coherence tomography); Carl Zeiss Meditec has detected sectorial thinning of both eyes (**Figure 9**).

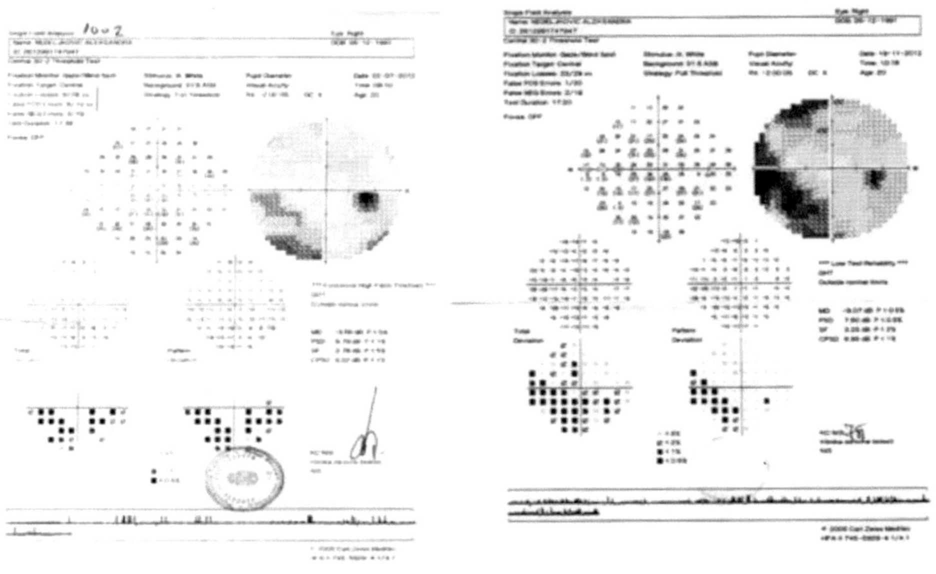

Figure 4. SAP of the right eye (VII/XI 2012) OD: relative paracentral visual field defects (MD = −9.07 dB; CPSD = 6.65 dB).

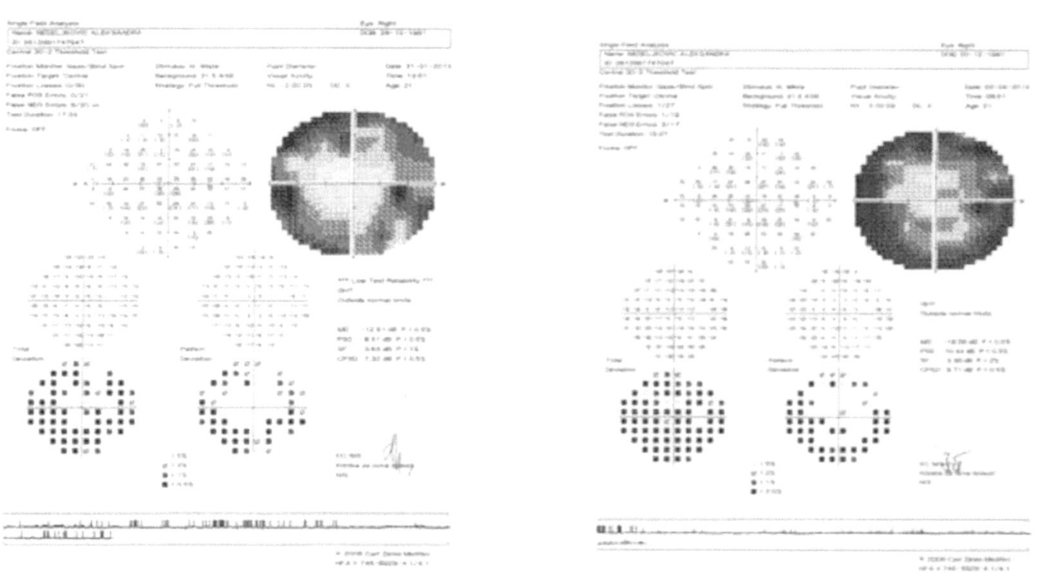

Figure 5. SAP of the right eye (I/IV 2013) OD: constriction of the visual field (MD = −18.56 dB; CPSD = 9.71 dB).

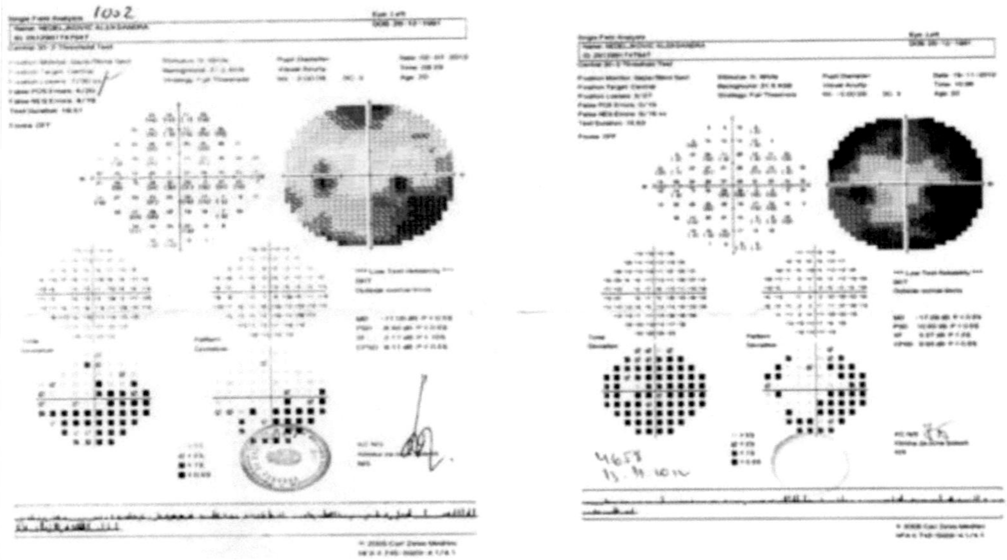

Figure 6. SAP of the left eye (VII/XI 2012) OS: blind spot enlargement, relative and absolute paracentral visual field defects (MD = −17.28 dB; CPSD = 9.93 dB).

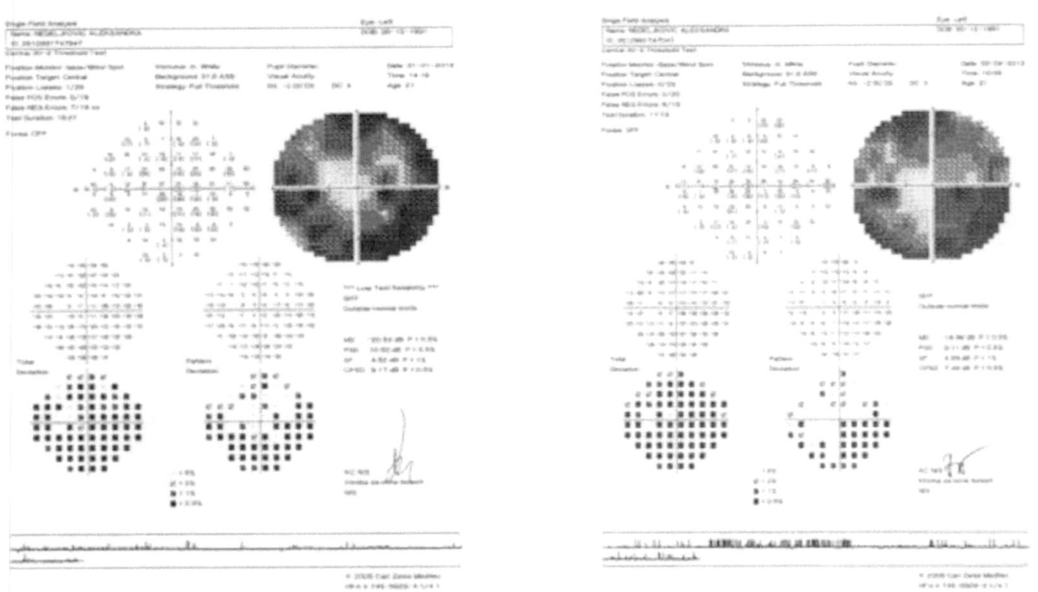

Figure 7. SAP of the left eye (I/IV 2013) OS: narrowing of the visual field up to 10°, inferior nasal quadrantanopia (MD = −18.96 dB; CPSD = 7.48 dB).

The electrophysiological examination recorded regular answers of parameters, prolonged latency of the P100 wave in the right eye (OD: P100 = 117 ms; OS: P100 = 113.7 ms).

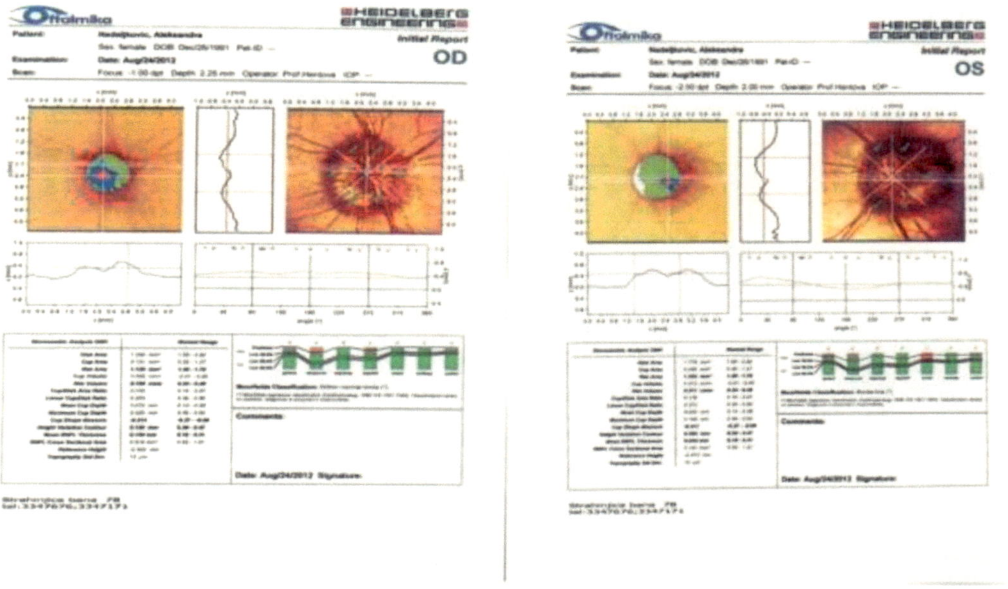

Figure 8. HRT (VIII/2012) OD: DA = 1256; mean RNFL = 0.130; OS: DA = 1778; mean RNFL = 0.034.

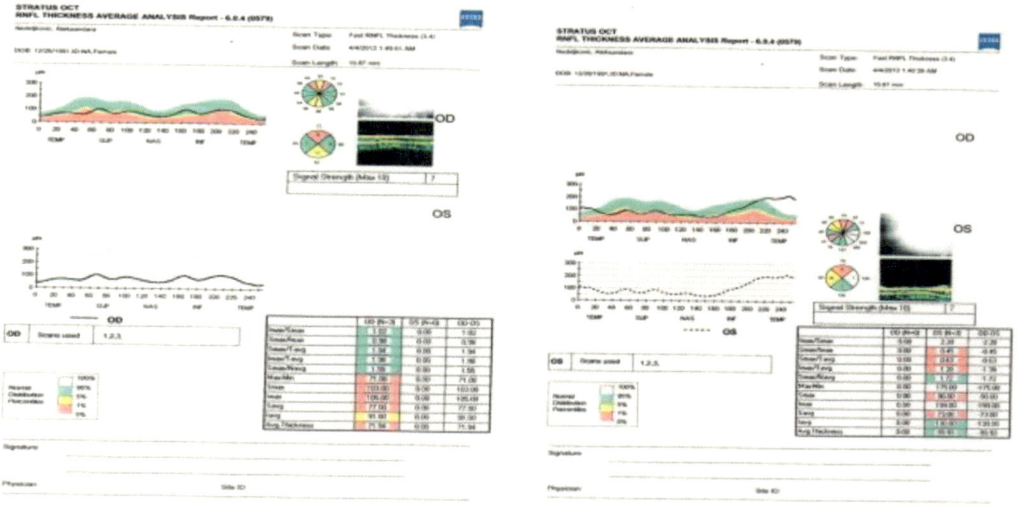

Figure 9. OCT (stratus 6.0.4. IV/2013) RNFL OD: Savg = 77.0, Iavg = 91.0, Navg = 66.0, and Avg thick = 71.94. RNFL OS: Savg = 73.0, Iavg = 130.0, Navg = 53.0, and Avg thick = 93.93.

Computerized tomography (CT) of the endocranium and the orbit on an axial scan showed bilateral calcification at the ONH (**Figure 10**).

Six months after topical hypotensive drug administration, an improvement of the visual field resulted in the improvement of reduced sensitivity. Depth and extensions of the scotomas were improved and maintained during the monitoring period of at least 3 years. The finding was also confirmed by the last visual field testing (**Figures 11** and **12**).

Relative and absolute paracentral and peripheral scotomas are still present, partly confluent, more in the nasal periphery of the left eye.

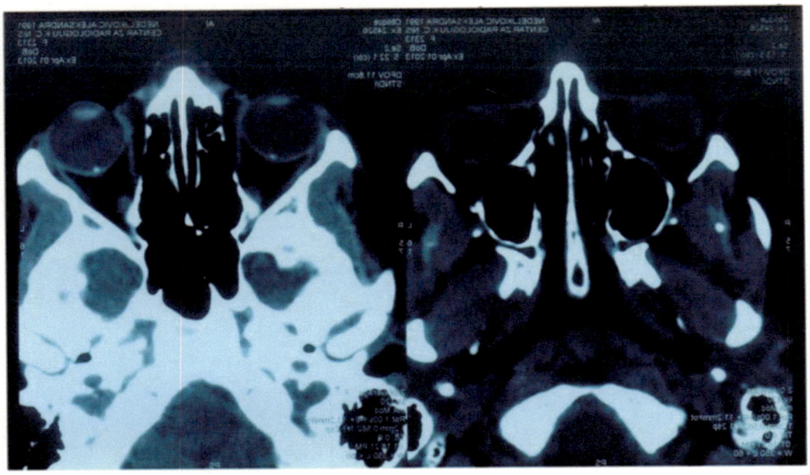

Figure 10. CT (IV/2013) No pathological changes in the endocranium. Bilateral calcification at the ONH.

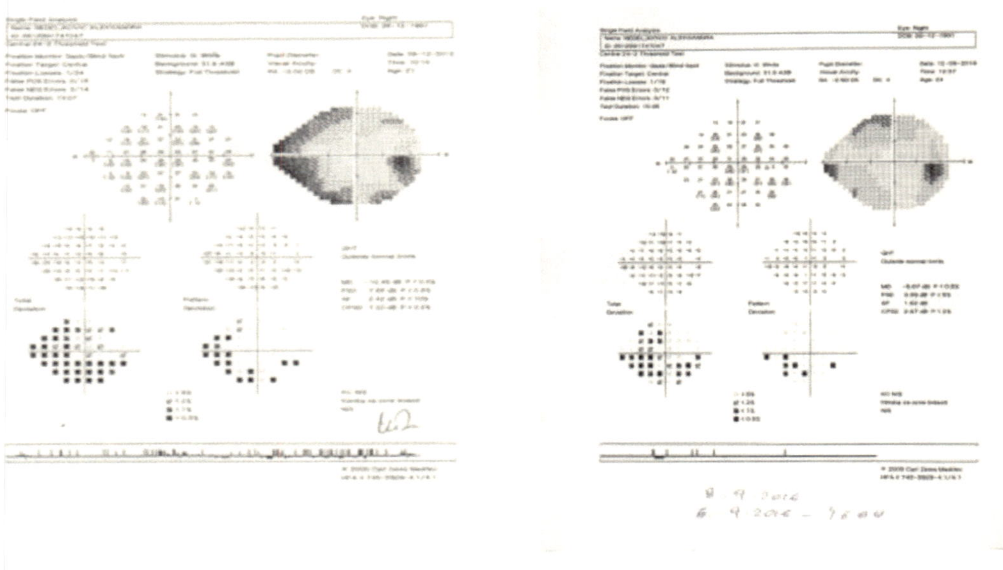

Figure 11. SAP of the right eye after therapy introduction: KP(XII/2013) OD: MD = −10.46 dB; CPSD = 7.20 dB; KP (IX/2016) OD (MD = −6.67 dB; CPSD = 2.97 dB).

http://dx.doi.org/10.5772/intechopen.80278

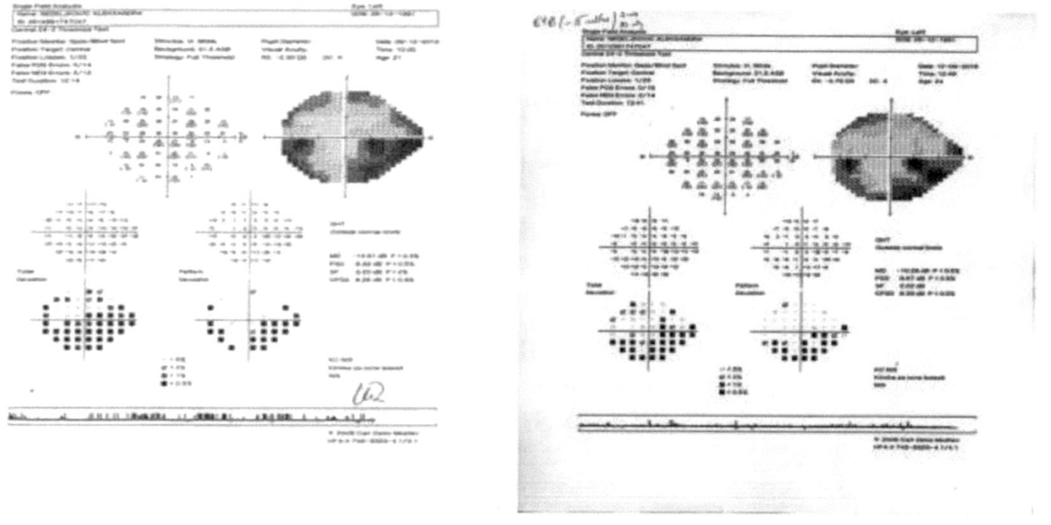

Figure 12. KP of the left eye after therapy introduction: KP(XII/2013) OS: MD = −13,51 dB; CPSD = 8,25 dB); KP (IX/2016) OS (MD = −10.28 dB; CPSD = 8.39 dB).

3. Discussion

A young female patient with advanced visual field defects because of the ONH drusen is presented. Visual field defect is one of the most common drusen complications in these cases with preserved central visual acuity. Although a patient has myopic refraction, it was concluded that the disk area is smaller (based on HRT). That was more pronounced on the right eye (OD: DA = 1.256 mm^2; OS: DA = 1.778 mm^2) when compared to the normative values of 1.69–2.82 mm^2. That indicated how a small diameter of the scleral canal can compromise axoplasmic transport. The conclusion of one of the conducted studies suggested that the incidence of drusen is greater if DA is smaller than 1.79 mm^2, with a confidence interval of $p < 0.001$. There is also confirmation that drusen are present in more than 50% of patients with a small horizontal diameter of the optic nerve head (1.68 ± 0.18 mm). Different authors agreed that the chronic obstruction of axoplasmic transport due to the small diameter of the scleral canal results in drusen formation [10, 26].

There are three basic theories in explaining pathogenesis of drusen:

1. Degenerative axonal death (Seitz)
2. Protein transudation from congenitally abnormal vessels of the disk (Sacks)
3. Alteration of axoplasmic transport (Spenser)

The slowly progressive visual field loss is characteristic of the drusen (Lauber) as a result of a direct mechanical compression followed by axonal dysfunction and degeneration. The incidence of scotomas, as one of the most common complications of optic nerve drusen, is 24–87% in adults with a progression rate of 1.6% per year. Visual field defect may occur even in childhood [11, 27]. The rule in appearance, depth, duration, and the type of scotoma was not determined. The most common are peripheral, arcuate scotoma, enlargement of the blind spot, rarely the nasal step, and generalized constriction of the visual field. Scotomas are variable depending on the grade of drusen. In severe cases, they become confluent to inferonasal quadrantanopia to hemianopia [27, 28]. In the presented clinical case, an irregular incidence of scotomas was observed in relation to the grade of drusen (grade I in the right eye; grade II in the left eye). Savino et al. founded 71% of the visual field defects for visible drusen, compared to 21% in the case of hidden ones [14].

An attempt was made to correlate distribution of scotoma with localization and number of optic nerve drusen. In Grippo's retrospective study in 103 eyes was found that in superficial drusen (grade III), visual field defect was advanced, while in the case of hidden drusen (grade I), it was the initial, which was confirmed through this presentation. The distribution of scotoma often does not correspond completely with the localization of visible drusen, most likely due to the simultaneous presence of hidden ones and extensive axonal lesions [11]. Thus, there are scotomas with irregular distribution on the right eye of our patient with hidden drusen. Some of the reports noted 76.3% of scotomas in visible drusen compared to 46.5% in the case of hidden drusen [29, 30]. In the remaining half of patients with the first (I) grade of the drusen, in 5% of cases, an arcuate scotoma could be developed [31].

Any decrease in central visual acuity, rapidly progressive visual field loss, or arcuate scotoma in drusen requires careful consideration of the etiology in terms of glaucoma or neuro-ophthalmology background [11]. Concomitant drusen and glaucoma can cause extensive visual field damage, which can cause a diagnostic and therapeutic dilemma. It was found that the grade of drusen and IOP level directly, independently, and significantly correlate with the degree of damage of the visual field. The result is a unique attitude of introducing topical hypotensive therapy in both cases in the aim to reduce the risk of further damage [1, 16, 32].

Visual field damage occurs in 90.9% of hypertensive versus 66.7% of normotensive eyes. Higher IOP is statistically significantly associated with advanced impairments regardless of age, sex, and grade of drusen [11, 15]. In our case presentation of a young female patient, elevated IOP or association with glaucoma for the entire duration of follow-up period was not confirmed, which was confirmed by testing. Flame microhemorrhages that may occur at the RNFL in glaucoma have been observed, but not found. Hemorrhages are thought to have no effect on the occurrence of scotomas in drusen, opposed to numerous and confluent flame-shaped hemorrhages in the real existing edema of the optic nerve head. There are no major controlled clinical studies of the effects of topical hypotensive drugs in drusen, but there are numerous individual reports, as well as announcements of small sample of patients confirming the benefit of topical hypotensive drugs due to indirect enhancement of ONH perfusion (Grippo, Poda-Wilczek, Spalding, Patel, Czajor, Moris) [1, 4, 15, 18, 33–35].

Due to the extension and depth of the scotoma, as well as their progression over the monitoring period of 6 months, although the patient did not have an elevated IOP, after examination of the literature and actual reports, topical hypotensive therapy was applied. The first therapeutic choice was brimonidine 0.2% for 3 months, but after an allergic reaction, it was replaced with latanoprost 0.005% (due to patient age and frequency of drug application). There is no specific and precise recommendation about therapeutic choice. Most commonly carboanhydrase inhibitors are used.

In these cases, the decision to use medication was made after a regular CT and the exclusion of a potential neuro-ophthalmological disease (pseudotumor cerebri) and SAP findings (right eye, MD = −18.56 dB; left eye, MD = −18.96 dB). After 6 months, the depth of visual field defects was reduced (right eye, MD = −10.46 dB; left eye, MD = −13.51 dB).

An improvement in sensitivity reduction has been achieved, from the advanced to the initial (right eye)/moderate (left eye) stage, and was confirmed by the 1-year SAP and at the last SAP finding (IX/2016) (right eye, MD = −6,67 dB; left eye, MD = 10,28 dB).

In addition to functional, it is advisable to monitor structural damage by imaging techniques. Retinal nerve fiber layer (RNFL) thinning is a pathological finding detected in drusen, by using modern technologies: OCT (EDI-OCT), HRT, and laser scanning polarimetry (GDx) [9]. Roh et al. suggested OCT as a sensitive and confident method for the early detection of RNFL thinning in drusen and/or glaucoma [36, 37].

A combination of methods that confirm anatomical lesion (OCT) and functional impairment (SAP, electrophysiological testing) is necessary in making a right decision when and how to treat by topical hypotensive drugs [4]. Recent studies confirmed that OCT is a significant method in the differentiation of ONH drusen from the real edema of the ONH by means of qualitative and quantitative criteria [10]. Both entities are presented with elevation and unclear border of the ONH, and the qualitative criterion helps in the differentiation with a sensitivity of 63%, because in real edema, an internal contour line of the optic nerve is a straight line as well as the widened subretinal hyporeflective space (SHYPS), unlike in pseudoedema with the undulating line ("lumpy-bumpy" line) and with narrow SHYPS (Savini). The thickness of subretinal hyporeflective space (SHYPS) in edema is greater than 464 μm and in a diameter of 2 mm greater than 127 μm. Using EDI-OCT, it is possible to find out hidden drusen and their posterior border with a depth of 500–800 μm, deeper than a conventional OCT [38, 39].

The quantitative parameter is the measurement of RNFL thickness (total and sectoral) with a sensitivity of 90%, with a significant thinning before occurrence of scotoma in the visual field. RNFL thinning correlates with the scotoma location, but not always with the degree of damage of the visual field. The nasal sector is the predilection area [5]. Observed according to grades, I and II are dominant superiorly, while III is more frequent inferiorly [36]. Opposite to this, in ONH edema, the thickening of RNFL is observed [38]. The OCT findings of our patient show average and sectoral thinning, at superior sector in an eye with hidden drusen and nasally with superficial drusen, that correlates with previously mentioned observations. OCT angiography, with superficial laminar segmentation, usually shows focal capillary attenuation overlying the most prominent drusen. These findings demonstrate alterations in the superficial retinal capillary network associated with ONH drusen [40].

Heidelberg retinal tomography (HRT) provides three-dimensional topographic analysis of the ONH with the measurement of the height of the peripapillary RNFL that correlates with the changes in the visual field. Thus, the area of the ONH was analyzed, and the control HRT of our patient showed total RNFL thinning in the left eye 0.107 mm (0.18–0.31) [40, 41]. HRT is less sensitive than OCT in the RNFL estimation. It also shows anterior displacement of the cup bottom, in front of the RPE versus healthy subjects [40]. Polarimetric analysis of retinal nerve fibers (GDx) usually detects thinning, especially in the eyes with irregular and unclear ONH border and erased cupping [41–44]. In our patient it was not performed due to technical impossibility.

The retinal ganglion cell axons in the early phase of mechanical stress do not show immediate degeneration but enter the stage of functional disorder, presented with abnormal latency at the visual evoked potential (VEP) in more than 95% (Stevens). A minor clinical study of six patients with drusen but without symptoms showed prolonged P100 wave latency [11, 45]. More sensitive is the multifocal VEP (mf VEP) that allows the measurement of the latency of local VEP response from 60 sectors within the central 24° of visual field, which may be less evident on the standard VEP [46]. Grippo's analysis of patients with the drusen shows an altered finding in 28% of patients tested with conventional VEP and 70% of abnormal findings with mf VEP [15]. A careful review of the evoked potential of our patient shows a discretely prolonged P100 wave, more obvious in the right eye (right eye, 117 ms; left eye, 113.7 ms). That is a sign of initial dysfunction with normal visual acuity. In more affected eye, RAPD or reduction of amplitude N95 can be seen [9].

Vascular complications and abnormalities in patients with drusen are frequent also. They are caused by different mechanisms if they are associated with optic nerve head drusen. The most common cause of sudden visual loss may be non-arteritic anterior ischemic optic neuropathy (NAINO). Auw-Haedrich points out that people with drusen are more prone to ischemic attacks of the optic nerve head than those with a small diameter of the scleral canal and without drusen, because the arterial inflow becomes insufficient with their magnification. The younger age is more dominant among them in comparison to the years of life of patients with NAINO. CRAO, CRVO, and subretinal neovascularization adjacent to optic nerve head may also affect the younger population [2, 9]. Our patient did not have vascular complications because of the shorter duration of detected drusen and her age.

4. Conclusion

Young person with optic nerve head drusen is presented, the most common complications and performed findings of the diagnostic procedures that were carried out with the summarized current knowledge of epidemiology, pathogenesis, clinical presentation, diagnosis, and therapy of the eyes with optic nerve head drusen. Currently, there is no specific strictly indicated treatment and therapeutic protocol for the progressive damage of visual function and complications that may arise due to drusen. A preventive IOP reduction is recommended in order to reduce potential damage of the axons of the optic nerve [1]. The goal of the applied therapeutic concept was to reduce the IOP with the tendency of slowing down and stopping the progression of scotoma in the visual field, which is confirmed by the findings in this presentation and numerous pilot studies [1, 2]. Topical hypotensive drugs improve blood flow in the optic nerve head, thus reducing potential vascular damage due to the presence of drusen.

Following the correlation of years of life, the morphology of the optic nerve head, and the functional changes with drusen, it has been established that during the time, drusen can cause serious progressive optic neuropathy [47, 48]. The structural characteristics in the optic nerve head cause individual differences in the damages of retinal ganglion cell axons caused by intraocular pressure; therefore, lower IOP is recommended [49]. The importance of this, as well as other medical and surgical therapeutic modalities, especially neuroprotective drugs, is still being investigated in order to reduce potential morbidity.

Conflict of interest

The author declares no conflict of interest.

Thanks

My gratitude to Vladimir Radenkovic for the technical support.

Author details

Marija Radenković

Address all correspondence to: marad@verat.net; radenkovicmarija74@gmail.com

Eye Clinic, Clinical Center Nis, Serbia

References

[1] Morris RW, Ellerbrock JM, Hamp AM, Joy JT, Roels P, Davis CN Jr. Advanced visual field loss secondary to optic nerve head drusen: Case report and literature review. Optometry. 2009;**80**(2):83-100. DOI: 10.1016/j.optm.2008.11.004

[2] Schargus M, Gramer E. Optic disc drusen. Der Ophthalmologe. 2008;**105**(7):693-710. DOI: 10.1007/s00347-008-1762-7

[3] Auw-Haedrich C, Staubach F, Witschel H. Optic disk drusen. Survey of Ophthalmology. 2002;**47**(6):515-532. PMID: 12504737

[4] Czajor K, Misiuk-Hojło M. Heidelberg edge perimetry in optic nerve drusen—A case report. MEDtube Science. 2014;**II**(1):29-33

[5] Ubhi P, Shechtman D, Green K. Discern optic nerve head Drusen from true papilledema. Review of Optometry. 15 Dec 2015;**2015**:44-47

[6] Friedman AH, Henkind P, Gartner S. Drusen of the optic disc. A histopathological study. Transactions of the Ophthalmological Societies of the United Kingdom. 1975;**95**(1):4-9. PMID: 1064209

[7] Chang MY, Pineles SL. Optic disk drusen in children. Survey of Ophthalmology. 2016;**61**(6):745-758. DOI: 10.1016/j.survophthal.2016.03.007

[8] Gay D, Boyer S. Two differing presentations of optic nerve head drusen. Optometry. 2001;**72**(9):588-596. PMID: 11575696

[9] Davis PL, Jay WM. Optic nerve head drusen. Seminars in Ophthalmology. 2003;**18**(4):222-242. DOI: 10.1080/08820530390895244

[10] Gili P, Flores-Rodríguez P, Yangüela J, Orduña-Azcona J, Martín-Ríos M. Evaluation of optic disc size in patients with optic nerve head drusen using fundus photography. Journal of Optometry. 2013;**6**(2):75-79

[11] Grippo TM, Rogers SW, Tsai JC. Optic disc drusen. Glaucoma Today. Jan/Feb 2012;**2012**:19-24

[12] Gaillard F. Optic Disc Drusen. 2005-2017. Available from: http://radiopaedia.org

[13] Aumiller MS. Optic disc drusen: Complications and management. Optometry. 2007;**78**(1): 10-16. DOI: 10.1016/j.optm.2006.07.009

[14] Jonas JB, Gusek GC, Guggenmoos Holzmann I, Naumann GO. Pseudopapilledema associated with abnormally small optic discs. Acta Ophthalmologica. 1988;**66**(2):190-193. PMID: 3389093

[15] Grippo TM, Shihadeh WA, Schargus M, Gramer E, Tello C, et al. Optic nerve head drusen and visual field loss in normotensive and hypertensive eyes. Journal of Glaucoma. 2008;**17**:100-104. DOI: 10.1097/IJG.0b013e31814b995a

[16] Kamjoo S, Epley KD, Pihlbad MS. Optic Disc Drusen. 2015. Available from: http://eyewiki.aao.org

[17] Gossman MV. Pseudopapilledema. 2015. Available from: http://emedicine.medscape.com

[18] Patel V, Oetting TA. Optic Nerve Drusen: 19-year-old Female with Blurred Vision. EyeRounds.org. 2007. Available from: http://www.EyeRounds.org/cases

[19] Sadun AA, Wang MY. Funduscopic features. In: Handbook of Clinical Neurology. Vol. 102. New York, United States: Elsevier; 2011. pp. 2-524

[20] Lyons CJ, Wiwatwongwana A. Pediatric neurology part III. The optic nerve and visual pathways. In: Handbook of Clinical Neurology. Vol. 113. New York, United States: Elsevier; 2013. pp. 1515-1525

[21] Delyfer MN, Rougier MB, Fourmaux E, Cousin P, Korobelnik JF. Laser photocoagulation for choroidal neovascular membrane associated with optic disc drusen. Acta Ophthalmologica Scandinavica. 2004;**82**(2):236-238. DOI: 10.1111/j.1600-0420.2004.00231.x

[22] Haritoglou C, Prieglinger SG, Grueterich M, Kampik A, Kriegelstein GK. Radial optic neurotomy for the treatment of acute functional impairment associated with optic

nerve drusen. The British Journal of Ophthalmology. 2005;**89**(6):779-780. DOI: 10.1136/bjo.2004.060335.

[23] Pfriem M, Hoerauf H. Unsuccessful surgical excision of optic nerve drusen. Graefe's Archive for Clinical and Experimental Ophthalmology. 2011;**249**(10):1583-1585. DOI: 10.1007/s00417-011-1693-x

[24] Kapur R, Pulido JS, Abraham JL, Sharma M, Buerk B, Edward DP. Histologic findings after surgical excision of optic nerve head drusen. Retina. 2008;**28**(1):143-146. DOI: 10.1097/IAE.0b013e31815e98d8

[25] Pinxten I, Stalmans P. Radial optic neurotomy as a treatment for anterior ischemic optic neuropathy secondary to optic disc drusen. GMS Ophthalmology Cases. 2014. DOI: 10.3205/oc000018

[26] Jonas JB, Gusek GC, Guggenmoos-Holzmann I, Naumann GO. Optic nerve head drusen associated with abnormally small optic discs. International Ophthalmology. 1987;**11**(2):79-82. PMID: 2451648

[27] Wilkins J, Pomeranz H. Visual manifestations of visible and buried optic disc drusen. Journal of Neuro-Ophthalmology. 2004;**24**(2):125-129. PMID: 15179065

[28] McCafferty B, McClelland CM, Lee MS. The diagnostic challenge of evaluating papilledema in the pediatric patient. Taiwan Journal of Ophthalmology. 2017;**7**(1):15-21. DOI: 10.4103/tjo.tjo_17_17

[29] Calvo-González C, Santos-Bueso E, Díaz-Valle D, Reche-Frutos J, Moriche-Carretero M, Benítez-Del-Castillo JM, et al. Optic nerve drusen and deep visual fields defects. Archivos de la Sociedad Española de Oftalmología. 2006;**81**(5):269-273. PMID: 16752318

[30] Obuchowska I, Mariak Z. Visual field defects in the optic disc drusen. Klinika Oczna. 2008;**110**(10-12):357-360. PMID: 19195165

[31] Katz BJ, Pomeranz HD. Visual field defects and retinal nerve fiber layer defects in eyes with buried optic nerve drusen. American Journal of Ophthalmology. 2006;**141**(2):248-253. DOI: 10.1016/j.ajo.2005.09.029

[32] Spalding JM. Visual-field loss with optic nerve drusen and ocular hypertension: A case report. Optometry. 2002;**73**(1):24-32. PMID: 12363235

[33] Sowka J, Kabat A. IOP, drusen and occlusion. Review of Optometry. 2016;**31**:118-119

[34] Pojda-Wilczek D, Herba E, Jedrzejewski W, Pojda SM. Optic disc drusen and glaucoma—Case report. Klinika Oczna. 2004;**106**(1-2 Suppl):263-265. PMID: 15510520

[35] Ziak P, Jarabáková K, Koyšová M. Optic disc drusen—Current diagnostic possibilities. Ceská a Slovenská Oftalmologie. 2014;**70**(1):30-35. PMID: 24862373

[36] Roh S, Noecker RJ, Schuman JS. Evaluation of coexisting optic nerve head drusen and glaucoma with optical coherence tomography. Ophthalmology. 1997;**104**:1138-1144. PMID: 9224467

[37] Roh S, Noecker RJ, Schuman JS, Hedges TR, Weiter JJ, Mattox C. Effect of optic nerve head drusen on nerve fiber layer thickness. Ophthalmology. 1998;**105**:878-885. DOI: 10.1016/S0161-6420(98)95031-X

[38] Johnson LN, Diehl ML, Hamm CW, Sommerville DN, Petroski GF. Differentiating optic disc edema from optic nerve head drusen on optical coherence tomography. Archives of Ophthalmology. 2009;**127**(1):45-49. DOI: 10.1001/archophthalmol.2008.524

[39] Silverman AL, Tatham AJ, Medeiros FA, Weinreb RN. Assessment of optic nerve head drusen using enhanced depth imaging and swept source optical coherence tomography. Journal of Neuro-Ophthalmology. 2014;**34**(2):198-205

[40] Gaier ED, Rizzo JF, Miller JB, Cestari DM. Focal capillary dropout associated with optic disc drusen using optical coherence tomographic angiography. Journal of Neuro-Ophthalmology. 2017;**37**(4):405-410. DOI: 10.1097/WNO.0000000000000502

[41] Pihlbad MS. Optic Nerve Head Drusen. 2015. Available from: http://eyewiki.aao.org

[42] Kuchenbecker J, Wecke T, Vorwerk CK, Behrens-Baumann W. Quantitative and objective topometrical analysis of drusen of the optic nerve head with the Heidelberg retina tomograph (HRT). Der Ophthalmologe. 2002;**99**(10):768-773. DOI: 10.1007/s00347-002-0639-4.

[43] Patel NN, Shulman JP, Chin KJ, Finger PT. Optical coherence tomography/scanning laser ophthalmoscopy imaging of optic nerve head drusen. Ophthalmic Surgery, Lasers & Imaging. 2010;**41**(6):614-621. DOI: 10.3928/15428877-20100929-07

[44] Tatlipinar S, Kadayifcilar S, Bozkurt B, Gedik S, Karaagaoglu E, Orhan M, et al. Polarimetric nerve fiber analysis in patients with visible optic nerve head drusen. Journal of Neuro-Ophthalmology. 2001;**21**(4):245-249. PMID: 11756852

[45] Vieregge P, Rosengart A, Mehdorn E, Wessel K, Kömpf D. Drusen papilla with vision disorder and pathologic visual evoked potentials. Der Nervenarzt. 1990;**61**(6):364-368. PMID: 2377263

[46] Grippo TM, Ezon I, Kanadani FN, Wangsupadilok B, Tello C, Liebmann JM, et al. The effects of optic disc drusen on the latency of the pattern-reversal checkerboard and multifocal visual evoked potentials. Investigative Ophthalmology & Visual Science. 2009;**50**(9):4199-4204. DOI: 10.1167/iovs.08-2887

[47] Schargus M, Grippo T, Ritch R, Gramer E. Stage of visual field loss in relation to the appearance of the optic disc in 144 eyes of patients with drusen of the optic disc. Investigative Ophthalmology & Visual Science. 2005;**46**:2483

[48] Tanaka H, Shimada Y, Nakamura A, Tanikawa A, Horiguchi M. A case of bilateral optic nerve head drusen-induced inferior altitudinal hemianopsia. Neuro-Ophthalmology. 2015;**39**(4):201-206. DOI: 10.3109/01658107.2015.1022899

[49] El-Assal K, Tatham AJ. Rapidly progressing visual loss associated with optic nerve head drusen: Is there a role for lowering intraocular pressure? Journal of Ophthalmic Science. 2016;**1**(2):23-33. DOI: 10.14302/issn.2470-0436.jos-15-763